Heartfelt

Caregiver's Guide to Cardiomyopathy and Mitral Valve Surgery

Elaine Webster

Books by Elaine Webster

Jesse's Tale
Overcoming Fear Aggression and Separation Anxiety in an Adopted Greyhound

Table of Contents

Acknowledgments

To say this book wouldn't have been possible without my husband Blake seems jocular, especially given the subject matter. Aside from his obvious contribution to this book, he plays the role of leading man in my life and is paramount to my success as a person and a writer. He is my best friend and steadfast partner. The happy ending to this book has opened a new chapter in our lives—both on and off these pages.

Steve Boga, my editor, friend, and writing coach, has opened doors that I'd never have gone through on my own. It is through his encouragement that I continue to grow as a writer. His editing work greatly improved this book.

Not long after I met Steve, I introduced him to Blake. The two men are now friends and business partners. This book is self-published through their joint venture, Media Design Publishing (www.mediadesignpublishing.com). I am particularly grateful to them for supporting this effort, from inception to publication.

Blake designed the cover and the book's website (www.heartfeltcaregiversguide.com).

Introduction

We've seen impressive advances in the treatment of heart disease over the past twenty or so years. What was once considered a death sentence is now often curable. This is especially true with valve-repair and replacement surgeries.

My husband Blake's mitral valve was damaged as a result of a childhood bout with rheumatic fever. He lived with few repercussions until his midforties, when his overworked heart became enlarged and he was diagnosed with cardiomyopathy. This is where my story begins.

In this book you will follow us through two surgically implanted ICDs (Inplantable Cardiac Defibrillators), twelve years of medication therapy, and finally open-heart surgery to repair the mitral valve. The result? Blake has never felt better.

I wrote this book with a heart patient's caregiver in mind. I offer you both practical advice and genuine reassurance. I show you how I coped with stress and stayed strong but also share the times I fell apart—and how and where I found comfort. It is a personal journey, made public, to help others who will follow.

As caregiver, you and your patient will rely on many medical providers. With two exceptions, Blake and I had positive experiences with our medical people. In those two instances, names have been changed.

Chapter One
The First Episode

Life's a Beach

My husband, Blake, has a big heart. From a philosophical, spiritual, and romantic viewpoint, this is a good thing. From a physical standpoint—not so good.

It was our twenty-fifth wedding anniversary, April 19, 1999. On the road to Gualala, a picturesque town on the rugged northern California coast, we stopped for a picnic lunch at our favorite beach. Blake had been congested for weeks; we assumed it was allergies, for which Sonoma County is notorious. We snacked on smoked salmon, havarti cheese, fruit, and sourdough bread. Afterward, as we were loading the beach chairs and ice chest into the back of our truck, Blake's face suddenly went white and he fell to his knees.

"Honey, you okay?" I asked as I helped him to his feet.

"I don't know. I feel faint. Maybe it's the antihistamines I took earlier."

"Should you try some DayQuil?" I was still thinking that pollen was the culprit.

I found a decongestant and gave it to him with some water; it seemed to help. Blake's color returned to normal and his breathing evened out.

"How do you feel?"

"Okay . . . but that was weird. I don't remember ever feeling that way before. It's like I left my body for a moment."

"Should we go home?"

"No, no. I'm all right . . . I think. I'd hate to forfeit our reservations. Let's keep going and see how I feel."

In Gualala, we checked into our favorite room at The Breakers Inn—the French-themed Normandy room. The frilly four-poster bed beckoned and hoping the fresh sea air would relieve Blake's congestion, we went to bed early. I fell asleep; Blake didn't. Instead he lay awake fighting a suffocating panic.

In the morning, I opened my eyes and saw Blake seated upright in a chair, staring out at the ocean. "Are you okay, sweetie?" I asked. "Did you get any sleep?"

"No, I've been up all night. I had the feeling that if I drifted off to sleep, I'd never wake up again."

"That's it," I said, "We're going to the doctor."

We packed our bags and headed back to Santa Rosa, to our primary-care physician's office. Not used to driving Blake's pickup, I white-knuckled my way through the twists and turns of Highway 1 while Blake coughed and sneezed.

His pasty pallor got him an immediate audience with the doctor.

Dr. Devore, looking at his watch, entered the exam room. He was about to leave for vacation and it had been one delay after another all morning.

"Doctor, I can't seem to get a blood-pressure reading," the nurse said as she pumped the monitor to inflation a second time.

"Have I seen you before?" Dr. Devore looked at Blake, trying to place him. "I'm not taking any new patients."

The nurse interceded. "Blake hasn't been in for a few years, but we've located his chart."

In a seemingly accusatory tone, the doctor asked, "What drugs are you on? What did you take?"

"Nothing . . . really. I don't know what's going on," Blake insisted.

"Take your shirt off. I want to listen to your heart and lungs."

Blake complied, and after a few moments the doctor asked, "Do you know you have a heart murmur?"

"Since I was little. I had rheumatic fever as a child and it did something to my heart."

"Well, it's probably the root of your problem, but I can't diagnose it. You'll need to see a cardiologist. Brenda at the front desk will get you an appointment before you leave today. Meanwhile, I'll give you a prescription for a beta blocker, which should help with the arrhythmias. I'm sorry, that's the best I can do today."

Diagnosis

The next morning, I returned to work and Blake met with Dr. Gregory, a cardiologist. An initial exam and echocardiogram diagnosed the problem, cardiomyopathy—an enlarged heart and a leaking mitral valve. An angiogram and a Medtronic Cardiac Defibrillator implant were scheduled at Santa Rosa Memorial Hospital for the following week.

"The arrhythmia you had was serious," the doctor told Blake. "In fact, I'm surprised you survived it at all. I want you to take it easy until we put in the implant. The beta blocker should help, but there's no guarantee that you won't have another episode. Meanwhile, I want you on a low sodium-diet."

"Well, we already eat well and don't add salt to anything," Blake said.

Dr. Gregory, with a full waiting room of elderly heart patients, looked absentmindedly at his watch. "Look, the girls up front will give you a list of what to eat . . . anything else?" And he was gone.

Blake stared at the open exam-room door for a few seconds, then made his way back to the front desk.

"Excuse me," he stammered.

"Yes?" answered the receptionist, her eyes glued to her computer screen.

"The doctor said you'd give me some dietary information?"

"Gail, could you get Mr. Webster our standard info packet?" she shouted, never looking at Blake.

Another young woman handed Blake a brown manila folder, turned her back, and went back to her desk. Blake stood for a moment, expecting something else—a kind word, some reassurance. Feeling awkward, he turned to leave just as the nurse called the next patient.

On his way home, he dropped by Dr. Devore's office. Brenda greeted him with a smile, his first of the day. "Hi, Blake. Back so soon?"

"I don't have an appointment, but was wondering if I could talk to Dr. Devore for a minute."

"Hold on a second," she said. "I think he just finished with a patient."

A moment later, Blake was sitting across the desk from Dr. Devore. "So, how'd it go with Dr. Gregory?" the doctor asked.

"Okay, I guess. But I was wondering if you could refer me to someone else."

"Look, Blake, I already know what you're going to say—no one likes Dr. Gregory's not-so-charming personality. But I really think he's the best choice right now. Of all the local cardiologists, he's known for his aggressive treatment and believe me, he's extremely competent."

"I trust your judgment, but I'm nervous that he's missing something. He's so abrupt," Blake argued.

"Well, he's prescribed appropriate medications, scheduled hospital time, and set follow-up appointments every three months for the next year. What else do you think you need?"

"I guess, nothing, except some courtesy."

"Well courtesy won't help your heart. Only good medical care will do that."

* * * *

That evening, Blake dropped a file folder on the kitchen counter. "Here's what they gave me at the cardiologist's office today."

I dried my hands on a dishtowel and flipped through the handouts. "What about these sodium levels? I have no idea what's considered high."

"They said to check the labels and try not to eat anything over 150 milligrams per serving. Ideally I shouldn't be eating more than 1000 milligrams per day." Blake grabbed a jar of pasta sauce from the cupboard.

"How much does that have?" I asked.

Blake put on his reading glasses and stared at the label. "A thousand milligrams per cup."

"Let me see that." I examined the label and sure enough, one serving provided all the salt Blake should have in a full day.

We scoured the kitchen cabinets and refrigerator shelves, scrutinizing labels. We had assumed that if we avoided the saltshaker Blake's sodium intake would be fine. Not true—anything in a jar, package, or can was loaded with salt. By the time we finished our search-and-destroy mission, we had filled four boxes and several bags for the local food bank.

"So, what are we going to have for dinner? We're cleaned out," Blake said.

"Well, not entirely. There's still fresh fruit, vegetables, grains, poultry, and fish." I picked up a package of spaghetti. "Look, pasta is zero milligrams. We'll start here."

Emergency

The near-death experience, still fresh on Blake's mind, had us afraid to leave the house. Every sneeze, cough, and heart flutter caused concern. Then, on the Saturday before the scheduled implant surgery—another attack. From my upstairs home office, I heard a crash resonate from Blake's office. I rushed down the hall to find him once more on his knees, a broken lamp nearby. Shaking, he looked up at me.

"I'm afraid I'm not going to make it until Monday," he stammered.

"We're going to the emergency room, right now!" I announced.

Santa Rosa Memorial Hospital's waiting room was crowded, but Blake's ghostly pallor again got us right in. I filled out the admittance and insurance forms while the orderlies helped Blake out of his clothes and into a hospital gown. By the time I reached his bedside, the attending doctor had admissions calling for a bed upstairs.

"He's too unstable," the attending physician said. "We can't let him leave. There's no way to know when he'll have another episode, and the next one could be fatal. I see he's scheduled for an implant on Monday. It's best if he stays here for the weekend."

Nodding, I accompanied my husband upstairs.

"I feel so stupid being here," Blake said a few minutes later. He was sitting on the edge of the hospital bed; the color had returned to his face. "I feel fine now."

"I know, but we can't take any chances." I gazed out at the parking lot below. "At least you have a window."

He did not, however, have a private room. In the bed near the door lay a semiconscious man who tossed, turned, and moaned incessantly.

"It could be worse . . . you could be him." I gestured toward the divider curtain.

"I wonder what's wrong with him," Blake said.

"I don't know, but it sounds painful."

From behind the curtain we heard a woman's voice. "My husband had part of his colon removed."

"Oh, I'm sorry, I didn't see you there," I said awkwardly.

"No problem. I think I nodded off . . . neither of us got much sleep last night. The nurses increased his morphine, but it didn't help much. He cried most of the night."

"You spent the night here?" I asked.

By this time she was standing by the curtain. She brushed her blond bangs from her forehead, revealing a flawless complexion except for the dark circles under her eyes. I guessed her to be in her late forties or early fifties.

"What's wrong with you?" she asked Blake. "You look so healthy."

To break up the boredom, we told our story. After we chatted for several minutes, she asked if we had an Advanced Health Care Directive: a legal document that would give me power of attorney to make healthcare decisions for Blake if he couldn't speak for himself. It covers medical treatment, choices of physicians, personal-care instructions, end-of-life decisions, and funeral arrangements.

"You really need to take care of that, especially with unstable arrhythmias," she urged.

"I know," I said. "But it's not legal without a witness and our friend who promised to come today flaked out. Blake's brother was here, but he can't witness it because he's a relative. So, I guess we'll have to take care of it later, when we get out."

"Look, I know you don't know me, but I can't tell you how important it is to have your wishes known before a procedure. You don't want a medical board deciding things if something goes wrong. Same with organ donations—you need to decide what you want ahead of time. If you want, I'll get the forms downstairs, bring them up, and I'll witness them for you."

"You'd do that for us?" I said, touched by her gesture. "Thank you so much."

"No problem. I'll be right back."

Long Days and Nights

"Zenith! There, I used my z and it's *Triple Letter Score*. That gives me thirty-seven points." I playfully stuck out my tongue at him and added my score to the *Scrabble* score sheet.

"Wait," Blake protested. "Isn't that a brand of TV set? You can't use proper names."

"Zenith, it means the highest point," I argued.

"I challenge."

"Again? Those challenges haven't worked out for you, and this will be no different." I opened my Webster pocket dictionary, found the page, and read: "Zenith: culmination, peak, summit. See, smarty pants . . . I win again."

Blake's look soured and he grabbed for the remote control. "I've lost six games of Scrabble in two hours. That's enough. I wonder what's on the tube."

As Blake clicked through the TV channels, a candy-striper stuck her head in the doorway. "Visiting hours are up . . . give him a kiss . . . it's time to go," she said as she skipped away to the next open door.

Blake and I said our goodbyes for the night, and I grabbed my purse and jacket. Back in the car, I shivered, although it was a warm May evening. *What a way to spend a Saturday night—alone.* I couldn't remember the last time we hadn't slept side-by-side.

As I stepped into our entryway, I was struck by the tomb-like silence. *Stop thinking of death*, I scolded myself. *He's going to be all right.*

I went through the house turning on lights, then pulled a wine glass from the cupboard and filled it to the brim from the open bottle of Zinfandel that Blake and I had started the night before. I balanced the full glass in one hand and hit another wall switch to illuminate the staircase. At the top of the stairs, I turned on every light in every room, plugged the bathtub and ran the water as hot as I could stand. While the tub filled, I booted my computer. The familiar opening chime of *Microsoft Windows* made me feel less alone. I had a connection.

Bath time over, I was glad for the bright lights as I opened a second bottle of wine. I thought about pouring a glass, then decided to take the bottle upstairs. Sleep was out of the question. I sat down at my computer and stared.

What did I know about all of this defibrillator stuff, anyway? My fingers took to the keyboard. For hours I researched. I found a website called *The Zappers*. Under the FAQs I learned that Zappers are people with defibrillator implants. There are two types of Zappers: *Joeys*, who have never been shocked, and *Electric Kangaroos* because they hop when shocked. At this point, slightly drunk, I found myself giggling.

I looked at the clock: 2:00 a.m. Still not sleepy, I started long emails to the seven people in my email address book. Six were friends, four of whom I hadn't seen in years, and one was my sister. I described what had happened, where Blake was, and what he was facing on Monday. To my sister, I confessed to feeling scared and lonely. We'd had little contact in the past six years, but the wine bolstered my courage. By the time I finished, tears blurred my vision and dripped on the keyboard. I expressed sadness for the insurmountable distance between us and tried to explain the reasons I left home—topics previously avoided. I had little faith that she would understand. Yet, I thought, *what the hell*, and hit the send button.

Finally at 4:00 a.m., I stumbled to bed. I couldn't see Blake until ten, and then it would be another full day of *Scrabble* and TV. I drifted off for four hours, tossing and turning, until streaks of sunlight hit my face through the blinds.

Testing, Testing, 1 2 3

"Double latté, please," I said to the clerk behind the coffee stand. I'd gotten to the hospital early Monday morning, prepared for a long day of waiting. Fueled with strong coffee, I rode the elevator to the second floor with a male orderly and an empty gurney. As we disembarked we headed in the same direction and ultimately to Blake's room.

“Time to go,” the gurney captain said as he pulled up next to Blake’s hospital bed.

I stepped aside, then noticed that Blake’s roommate was sitting up and smiling. He looked like a different person. His wife perched on the edge of his bed.

“Well, good morning,” I exclaimed. “You look great. How do you feel?”

“Well, I’ve been better, but the worst is over.”

“He’s going home tomorrow morning. Isn’t that great?”

“Cool.”

Just then Blake and the orderly rolled past me, and I had time only to wave an encouraging “thumbs up.” Memorial Hospital, as is now common in most hospitals, encourages caregivers to stay close to their loved ones. Gone are the days of isolated waiting rooms. I would follow Blake from one procedure to another—accessible and informed throughout the day. First stop, an angiogram.

In the hallway, before they wheeled him through the swinging doors, I gave Blake a kiss and a reassuring pat on the head. A wife’s role—one minute, lover; the next, mother. The small sunlit waiting room became my home for the next two hours. In a corner seat, an elderly woman, flipped through a *Sunset* magazine. In no mood to talk, I avoided her gaze. Instead, I spied a rack of informational brochures and snagged one on angiograms. I took it back to my carefully selected seat in the opposite corner.

The glossy three-fold pamphlet described an angiogram as an X-ray test that uses a special dye and camera (fluoroscopy) to take pictures of the blood flow in an artery (such as the aorta) or a vein (such as the vena cava). During an angiogram, a thin tube called a catheter is placed into a blood vessel in the groin (femoral artery or vein) or just above the elbow (brachial artery or vein). Then an iodine dye is injected into the vessel, making the area show up clearly in the X-ray pictures. This method is known as conventional or catheter angiogram. The angiogram pictures can be made into regular X-ray films or stored as digital pictures in a computer. The test's purpose is to find aneurysms (blood vessel bulges). It is also a search mission for narrow or blocked blood vessels that restrict blood flow. It is the main test for coronary artery disease.

Thanks to our healthy diet and exercise program, Blake sailed through the test—all channels clear. Next we moved to the Electrophysiology lab, where Dr. Chiang-Sing re-created an arrhythmia to see how easily Blake's heart when into "defib." I could tell by his facial expression as he approached me afterward in the waiting area that the news was not good. Apparently, Blake's heart needed very little coaching. Neither did we—we quickly agreed to go ahead with the implant.

An implantable cardioverter-defibrillator (often called an ICD) is a device that monitors and regulates the heartbeat. It is a surgically implanted pulse generator with one or more leads. A two-by-three-inch computer that runs on a battery, it directs electical charges through wires from the pulse generator to the inside of the heart. It's a two-way street. The unit administers the appropriate charges as it receives information back through the leads threaded into the heart.

Normally, a heart has a natural pacemaker (called the sinoatrial node) that helps your heart beat steadily. An electrical current starts in one of the upper chambers (the atria) and passes through the heart to the bottom chambers (the ventricles). Blake needed an ICD because of ventricular fibrillation (irregular heartbeat) and ventricular tachycardia (rapid heartbeat), which were causing his life-threatening arrhythmias. In fact, Blake had all the classic life-threatening symptoms—heart pounding, dizziness, and fainting.

During Blake's episodes, we were told, his heart quivered instead of beating. His blood flow stopped, and within seconds he passed out. Without an ICD to shock his heart, he'd die.

In people who don't have an ICD, ventricular fibrillation is treated with an external defibrillator. Paddles are placed on the chest, and the patient is electrically shocked. The heart then returns to a more normal rhythm. Blake would have his own personal paramedic implanted in his chest, and we were told to forget about calling 911, as this unit produced the same result.

An ICD constantly monitors heart rhythm. Programmed by the patient's doctor, it does several things:

- **Pacing**: It delivers pacing signals to help maintain a proper rhythm.

- **Cardioversion**: A shock is sent to the heart to stop a too-fast heartbeat.
- **Defibrillation**: If ventricular fibrillation is detected, it sends a stronger shock, helping the heartbeat return to normal.
- **Pacemaker**: When the heart beats too slowly, the ICD brings it up to normal.

The doctors assured us that most of the time Blake wouldn't even notice the device at work. Pacing produced a minimal sensation, a slight flutter. Cardioversion, however, depending on the strength of the shock, could feel like a mild thump in the chest. The defibrillator shock would be stronger still, more like a kick to the chest. It would come suddenly and last only a second. The upside is that it would save his life.

* * *

Blake came out of surgery with a small lump just below his collarbone. He awoke from the anesthesia without incident and by evening was resting comfortably. I sat at his bedside with a white binder and a three-hole paper punch balanced on the hospital tray table.

"I started a medical binder for you." I was in full-Virgo organizational mode. Blake just smiled and let me mother him. I handed him his sippy cup.

"From the information they gave me, it looks like you need to relax a few days, but then we're pretty much back to normal."

"I don't feel normal. I feel defective," he said. "Look at this lump in my chest. And what if the device goes off—what's it going to feel like to be shocked?"

"Oh, c'mon." I bent over and planted a kiss on his forehead. "We'll be all right."

"How do you know? I can't even talk to Gregory." Blake was referring to his cardiologist. "He acts like I'm stupid if I ask questions."

"Well, let's give it some time. I don't think it's a good idea to switch doctors so soon. If you still feel like that in a few months, we'll get a second opinion."

I stayed with Blake that evening until the nurses booted me out. Entering our empty house was less intimidating this time, requiring less light and less wine. I assured myself that Blake would be home the next day and we'd handle this together—just as we've always done.

Chapter Two
Live and Learn

Life Support—Finding the Right Doctor

Blake came away from his next appointment with Dr. Gregory with three prescriptions: Lanoxin to control atrial fibrillation (heart flutters), Lotensin to regulate blood pressure, and his miracle drug, Coreg. Coreg is a beta blocker, a drug that relaxes the heart so that it beats more efficiently. It also blocks the production of several harmful substances produced by the body in response to heart failure.

The aggressive drug therapy, although effective, had major side effects. Over the next four years, Blake complained incessantly about poor mental focus, dizziness, and fatigue. Each time, Dr. Gregory insisted that he stay the course and stop complaining. He also wanted Blake to take Lipitor, a drug to lower cholesterol, even though Blake's cholesterol readings were within the normal range.

"I don't understand," Blake said. "Why do I need to take one more drug?"

"For prevention," the doctor snapped.

"But you said my cholesterol levels are fine. Besides, I'm sticking to the low-fat, low-sodium diet, and I exercise."

"I really wish you'd let me be the doctor."

"Yeah, but look at this information sheet. Lipitor has its own side effects, like muscle aches, liver and kidney problems, and fatigue. If I get any more tired, I won't be able to do anything."

"Well, all right . . . all right . . . but I want you in here every three months for a cholesterol test. And I want you to consider surgery. That mitral valve needs replacement."

"Isn't that dangerous?" Blake was more scared and confused than ever.

"Anytime they crack your chest, it's dangerous. But would you rather die?"

Dr. Gregory did not like questions. Most of his patients were elderly and simply did as they were told, but Blake persisted.

"Aren't there any alternatives to what I'm taking?" As they talked, the Medtronic's Technician set up for a routine defibrillator check. The tiny room was cramped for three people.

Dr. Gregory dug in. "Listen, Blake, these side effects are normal and these are my preferred drugs."

Blake thought he noticed a concerned expression from the Medtronic's Technician. He tried to catch the man's eye, but he stayed focused on his portable computer screen.

"I'm doing a minor reset of the pacing," the technician said as he tapped on his computer touch screen. Can you feel that?"

"Yeah, slightly," Blake replied.

"Well, that's it for me," he said as he packed up. Blake thought he looked anxious to get out of there.

Dr. Gregory then set up for Blake's six-month echocardiogram—an ultrasound test that gives a clear picture of the heart on a computer screen. Several electrodes are attached to the patient and a clear gel is spread over the chest. An echo transducer records views of the heart. This safe and noninvasive test allows the doctor to check the size, shape, and strength of the heart. The heart valves are visible, and leakages are identified and measured.

"Is it supposed to make that noise?" Blake asked the doctor. "It seems awfully loud."

"Oh, it's fine . . . normal. Darn!"

"What's wrong?"

"Oh, this pedal keeps sticking . . . let me shift this around."

As Blake tried to lie still, Dr. Gregory pulled at the computer and the entangled wires. A pile of paperwork fell to the floor. "Damn it!" he muttered. "Here, get up a second and help me with this," he commanded.

Blake slid off the exam table, still tethered to the machine by electrodes. The two men gathered up the mess, and Blake helped untie several knotted computer cords. Finally, Blake climbed back onto the examination table and they finished the test.

* * * *

Blake continued to have trouble staying mentally focused. He had bouts of dizziness and fatigue. Uncomfortable speaking with his cardiologist, he tried to self-regulate his medications, so that he could work—bad idea. His blood pressure fluctuated from dangerously high to dangerously low. If he stood up suddenly, he'd feel faint. Finally I convinced him to call for an appointment. When he did, he asked the receptionist if it would help to bring his home blood-pressure readings with him to the office. She said yes.

On the day of his appointment, Blake took with him two weeks of charted blood pressure readings and a diary of side effects. After waiting an hour, he approached the receptionist and asked how much longer it would be.

"Oh, the doctor just called. He'll be here in another half hour. He had to stop at the fruit stand for apples."

Forty minutes later, the physician rushed in the door and past his waiting patients, with no apologies.

"Blake, Dr. Gregory will see you now," the nurse announced a few minutes later.

"So, Blake, why are you back so soon? Didn't I say to wait three months between appointments?" Dr. Gregory stared into Blake's file.

"Well, I'm not feeling well. I get dizzy and tired. And I want to know what to do—I can't function this way."

The doctor barely looked up from his chart. "Those reactions are completely normal. It takes time for your body to adjust to the medications."

"Well, I can't work because I have a hard time focusing . . . so I've been skipping dosages."

That got the doctor's attention. "I don't want you doing that. You have to follow the regimen I prescribed."

"Well, look." Blake held out the lists he'd brought.

"What are these?"

"I've been keeping track of my blood pressure at home and wrote down how I felt each day."

Dr. Gregory's face turned scarlet. He tossed the papers on the desk without even glancing at their contents. "These are worthless. I don't want you monitoring anything, that's my job."

Blake didn't know what to say. After a few seconds of awkward silence, Dr. Gregory, turned and walked away. Dumbfounded, Blake got dressed and left. He was in the parking lot when he heard his name called.

“Blake. Wait!” It was Dr. Gregory shouting from the medical building’s entrance. “Come back inside. I didn’t know they told you to bring these.”

Blake looked at his doctor waving the crumpled paperwork above his head. He hesitated, then with one last withering look at the doctor, climbed into his truck, turned over the engine, and drove away.

* * * *

A second visit with Dr. Devore got Blake two cardiologist referrals. One evening, as the aroma of Calamari Parmesan filled our kitchen, we pondered our choices over a glass of Cabernet Sauvignon from Amphora Winery.

“I Googled those two doctors, but didn’t find much about them,” I told Blake. “I also went to the Federation of State Medical Boards website (www.fsmb.org). For ten dollars per search I checked for disciplinary actions against both doctors—they were fine.”

“I know I need another cardiologist, but once I find one, I don’t want to have to change again. It’s too stressful.”

Just then the doorbell rang. It was our friend, Susan, bringing homemade Christmas cookies.

“Hey, guys, I’m just here to drop these off. What’s new?” Susan breezed into the kitchen and set her plate of sweets on the counter. She noticed the list of doctors.

“Lookin’ for a new cardiologist?”

“Yeah, I’ve had it with Gregory. I can’t talk to the guy.”

She pointed to one of the names on the list. “Well, this is the one you want. Dr. Erickson, he’s the best . . . everyone knows that. Cute too, not that it matters to you.”

With that, Susan hugged us both and flew back out the door, with a simple: “Merry Christmas, I’ll be in touch . . . got lots of deliveries to make tonight . . . ”

* * * *

“So, how’d it go with the new cardiologist?” I asked Blake as we sat down to dinner.

“Really good.”

Blake launched into a lengthy and enthusiastic description of his latest medical encounter. As I listened I thought about the pronounced differences between the two doctors. Dr. Erickson, it was clear, took the time to listen and answer questions. And unlike Dr. Gregory, he customized medical treatment to fit the patient. Rather than automatically prescribe the newest most-expensive drugs, he favored well-tested generics.

Blake was so much more engaged with Dr. Erickson. He no longer dreaded his appointments. With the doctor’s approval, he always took his medical binder, which I kept updated, our version of his medical history. He went to his appointments well prepared to ask questions, knowing they would be answered.

A Positive Patient Experience

We're often asked what constitutes a good doctor and how to tell if you have one. As in every human relationship the doctor-patient relationship is a partnership. Both sides must have common goals and be flexible. But what else? Blake and I put our heads together and came up with this list:

- **A clean, comfortable office**. A physician who cares about patients wants them to feel cared for from the moment they enter the office.
- **Friendly staff**. As the customer, you are entitled to be treated with respect and courtesy. Is it easy to get a live person on the phone when you call for an appointment, or with a question or concern?
- **Short waiting times**. Your time is as valuable as the physician's. An occasional unforeseen delay is understandable. If you regularly wait for an hour or more, it's a sign of an inefficient practice. If the well-dressed drug representative with the rolling suitcase is seen before you—and your appointment time has passed—it's a sign that the doctor considers the business end of medicine more important than your medical needs.
- **Modern up-to-date equipment**. Does your doctor utilize new technology? Does equipment appear well maintained?

▪ **Sufficient time**. Does the doctor schedule sufficient appointment time, so neither of you feels rushed? Can you talk to your doctor and are your concerns carefully considered and addressed?
▪ **Good communication**. Are treatment options, medication prescriptions, and medical procedures explained in a way you understand?
▪ **Personal connection**. Ideally, you are in partnership with your doctor and his or her staff. How do you feel when you have a doctor's appointment? Gut feelings are often right.

A Positive Physician Experience Demands:

▪ **Promptness and reliability**. Does the patient keep appointments, show up on time, and follow physician directions? Doctors and their staff are busy people. If you waste their time, you will not receive full attention. Remember that respect is a two-way street.
▪ **Preparation**. Does the patient come with an itemized list of questions? Are they, and any additional instructions, written down, either by the patient or an accompanying caregiver?
▪ **Good communication**. Is the patient pleasant, direct, and clear when speaking? If your doctor cringes every time your name appears on the appointment schedule, you are only hurting yourself. Don't be afraid to assert yourself, but stop short of becoming rude, demanding, or insulting.
▪ **Personal connection**. Most doctors go into medicine with a desire to help their patients. A likeable, cooperative patient is a pleasure to treat.

Blake Adjusts—Feeling Good and Moving Forward

Under the care of Dr. Erickson, Blake's attitude toward his health and well-being changed dramatically. Physician and patient worked together; by trial and error, they found the best medication regimen—one that Blake could tolerate without debilitating side effects. His energy levels still fluctuated, but the constant fatigue was gone. He could once again work and play effectively.

One look at Blake's cholesterol readings convinced Dr. Erickson that there was no need for Lipitor. "Your cholesterol is fine—no reason to test it so often. Now, let's figure out what to do about blood pressure. I do want you to keep it as low as possible, which will cut down on further mitral valve damage. Let's give Diovan a try."

"Dr. Gregory said I needed surgery to replace the valve. What do you think?" Blake asked apprehensively.

"I think it's premature. You may need surgery eventually, but for right now, let's get as much mileage out of this valve as possible. Nothing's better than original parts." The doctor smiled, and Blake let out a sigh of relief.

The biggest energy drain was the blood-pressure medications, of which there are many options. Eighty milligrams of Diovan once a day kept Blake's blood pressure around 100/60, low for the average person, but not so low that he felt dizzy.

With new-found oomph, Blake's creative juices began

flowing. He could work again, and he felt good about taking some pressure off of me, as primary caregiver.

"What ya looking at?" I asked one afternoon when I discovered Blake leafing through cookbooks.

"I'm getting tired of the same few meals we've come up with. I know you don't have much time to cook, so I thought I'd give it a try."

Though I had my doubts, I kept them to myself. In thirty years of marriage, I'd never seen Blake make more than a sandwich.

The next day I came home from work to the sound of swearing. "Damn it!"

"What's the matter?" I asked.

"There's something wrong with the oven. It won't heat up anymore."

"Let me see."

I fiddled with the dials and settings and sure enough, no heat. I pried what happened out of my husband. Blake had been heating water to cook lasagna noodles when he took a phone call; meanwhile, the pot boiled over. The stovetop burners were gas, but the oven was electric, and the hot water shorted out the computerized temperature regulator. Never fond of the stove that came with the house, we decided to go shopping.

Our Dream Stove—Healthy Heart Cooking

Asien's Appliance in downtown Santa Rosa is a kitchen Mecca. We spent a Saturday afternoon comparing basic gas ranges to the gorgeous stainless-steel professional models. We turned knobs, glided oven shelves in and out, read brochures, considered energy efficiency, but always returned to the same model, a 30-inch-wide, DCS five-burner wonder.

"I love this one, but it's so expensive," I said to Blake for the fifth time.

"My favorite, too," Blake agreed. "So, how do we rationalize the cost?"

"Hmm, how 'bout this? We've been married thirty years, we've never bought a new stove before, we're both going to use it to make you healthier, and it's the most beautiful thing I've ever seen. Oh, and did I tell you? . . . I love you."

The stove was delivered and installed the next weekend.

* * * *

Home Cooking

Blake's condition has taught us that restaurant food is laden with salt. This is true even in many vegan and vegetarian restaurants, which rely heavily on soy products, such as tamari (naturally fermented soy sauce) and miso (soup base), both high-sodium foods. Home cooking is the best way to insure that food is prepared with heart health in mind. If your family balks at the idea, remind them that low-salt, low-fat diets are best for everyone, not just heart patients. If you have young children, think about how you're helping them develop a taste for healthy cuisine. The medical profession now recognizes excess sodium as a contributor to a number of diseases. Americans have become so used to excess salt (40 percent of our food budget goes to eating out; one-third of kids eat salt-laden fast food daily) that lower sodium levels make food seem bland; however, once we get used to lower levels, it's salty foods that taste wrong.

Blake and I approached heart-healthy cooking with the same organizational skills we use in business. We sketched out a plan.

Menu

- Weekdays: Resolving to keep it simple, we made a list of our favorite quick and easy meals: burgers, grilled poultry and fish, pastas, salads, soups, and sandwiches.
- Weekends: Inspired by my favorite cooking shows and books, I agreed to spice things up on weekends. With imagination, a sense of adventure, and the right ingredients, it's easy to tweak recipes.
- Preparation: With only two of us, we divided meal preparation in half. If your family is larger, this is the perfect opportunity to involve everyone. Mutual support in difficult times cements families in new ways. And cooking is an act of love. Blake's efforts in the kitchen showed me that we were true partners in sickness and in health.

Grocery Shopping

- Supermarkets: Today, mainstream food companies recognize the need to lower salt levels in their products. Learn how to read labels. A good rule of thumb: Stay within the 150 to 200 milligrams per serving rule on any product.
- Fresh is best: Shop the outer edges of the store. Fresh meats, fish, fruits and vegetables are the best bets. Learn to cook from scratch, and enjoy simply prepared foods.
- Visit your local farmers' markets. Studies show that locally produced foods are more nutritious.
- Convenience foods: Stay away from prepared, packaged foods, even the ones that say "healthy." Read the sodium levels before you buy. I mostly avoid the frozen-food section.
- Mail order: For specialty items, such as condiments, soups, seasonings, and sauces, consider shopping online. Many hard-to-find, low- and sodium-free products can add flavor and diversity to everyday meals.
- Check out the recipes and the resource guide in the later chapters of this book for specific ideas and suggestions.

Tricks of the Trade—Kitchen Gadgets and Appliances

We have become masters of quick, easy, and flavorful food preparation. In lieu of salt we infuse flavor with herbs, spices, flavored vinegars and oils, wood-chip smoking, simple sauces, and innovative ingredient combinations. To make our job easier, we utilize a variety of appliances. A crock-pot meal thrown together the night before welcomes a hungry family home with enticing aromas. Summer barbeques bring friends and families together. A pizza stone produces a crust that equals any pizzeria. Food processors take the chore out of chopping and pureeing. You'll be amazed at what 15 to 20 minutes in the kitchen can produce.

Our Favorite Kitchen Helpers

- Slow cooker: For soups, stews, sauces, and chilis.
- Pressure cooker: To fast-cook almost anything, including dried beans.
- Food processor: Chop, grate, puree, and slice in seconds.
- Full-size and/or hand mixer: Mashed potatoes anyone?
- Bread machine: Does all the work for you. Homemade pizza dough never tasted so good.
- Barbeque: Ours is an outdoor propane version. Choose from a variety of quality indoor grills.
- Stovetop smoker. We found an inexpensive cast-aluminum version that smokes fish, chicken, and vegetables indoors in minutes. Our smoked fresh salsa has not a pinch of salt and plenty of flavor.
- Microwave: Shop any kitchen section for a myriad of microwave gadgets. There are vegetable steamers, egg cookers and even grills that work with your microwave to cook almost anything in minutes.
- Electric rice cooker: These inexpensive kitchen helpers allow you to "set it and forget it"—perfect rice every time.

Chapter Three
Quality Living

Exercise—Keep the Juices Flowing

A quality health club, with knowledgeable staff, good equipment, and friendly members is an excellent motivational tool for the heart challenged. Cardiologists agree that moderate strength training and consistent cardiovascular exercise is essential to good health. Armed with his doctor's approval, Blake scheduled an appointment with personal trainer, Jack Dixon, at the Airport Club in Santa Rosa.

"Let's start with a full health evaluation. Have a seat and I'll pull you up in the computer," Jack said after he welcomed his new client.

Ten minutes later, with Blake's vital statistics safely stored on the club's hard drive, the two men sketched out an exercise regiment. Blake had been an avid tennis player, but his medications made the hot courts unbearable. A strenuous match left Blake dehydrated from excess perspiration and exhausted from a lower-than-normal blood pressure. A climate-controlled, indoor workout made more sense.

"Because of your defibrillator placement, I don't recommend you push, pull, or lift more than fifty pounds," Jack said as he led Blake to the Cybex bench-press machine. "Let's start with thirty pounds and see how sore you are tomorrow."

At the end of the hour, Jack provided Blake with a personalized every-other-day exercise routine. For the first half hour, Blake rotated between weight machines, working different body parts. The second half of the hour he had his choice of cardio machines: treadmill, elliptical, stairsteppers, and bicycles. Within weeks Blake was in better shape than he'd been in years. And he'd fallen in love with yoga and qigong.

Popular Forms of Yoga and Qigong:

- Hatha yoga emphasizes core strength, posture, balance, flexibility, body alignment, and deep breathing. It's an excellent place to start if you've never exercised, or as a way to stretch and strengthen muscles fatigued from more strenuous exercise.
- Vinyasa yoga, more energetic, requires stamina, strength, balance, and mobility. You'll work up a sweat as you move through fluid poses in quick succession.
- Ashtanga and power yoga are more strenuous still. You will move quickly through a series of poses designed to build muscle and improve cardiovascular conditioning.
- Iyengar yoga is all about alignment. While using props, such as cushions, blankets, and blocks, poses are held for several minutes. Strengthened muscles become more flexible, and the inner organs of the body are stimulated and massaged. Blood flow increases and toxins dissipate.
- Qigong is a five-thousand-year-old mind-body healing art from China, the parent form of tai chi. The practice incorporates simple, deliberate movements that can be done standing or sitting. It focuses the mind and relaxes the body while improving strength and balance. The medical form of qigong is especially beneficial for the heart patient. Through visualization a person directs

qi—the life force—similar to the way acupuncture does it with needles. It is based on traditional Chinese medicine and although easy to learn, it requires a highly disciplined mind to achieve maximum results.

Emotional Support, Stress Control, and Meaningful Work

Blake and I follow the teachings of Paramahansa Yogananda, the Guru-Founder of Self Realization Fellowship (SRF) (www.yogananda-srf.org). The spiritual classic, *Autobiography of a Yogi*, chronicles his life and work. He founded SRF in 1920, and the organization continues with more than 500 temples, retreats, ashrams, and meditation centers around the world. The practice of kriya yoga, a meditation discipline, creates a foundation for spiritual progress. This is our path and I encourage you to find yours. A spiritual practice will give you emotional support through the most difficult physical challenges. Family and friends offer comfort, but not always at the exact time you need it—but God will. How you perceive your higher self is a personal choice. Whatever path you choose is bound to improve your health and well-being.

* * *

"Are you okay, honey?" I asked Blake one evening as I folded laundry. "You look nervous."

Blake stared blankly at me for a moment. "I can't get over the feeling of almost dying. I try to put it out of my mind, but it haunts me. The energy draining from my limbs,

Each time it happens, I think: *Oh no . . . not again . . . I can't take this anymore.*"

I pushed the piles of clothes aside and put my arms around my husband. "Yes, but you're still here and we're going to fix this thing. You will live to be an old man—you'll see."

Those few words and a warm hug were all Blake needed at that moment. That and a deep sigh and a stretch brought him back from despair. "Remember," I prompted, "in spite of the physical challenges, life should feel good and have balance. Undue stress will only add to the problem. Just yesterday, I read about a Benedictine monk, Bede Griffiths, who lived in India in the 1950s. His books urge people to live simply according to their religious values. He says that old age is the spiritual phase of life. The first two thirds of life prepare us for awakening of the spirit. For us this phase has begun—so, no fair checking out early and leaving me behind. Okay?"

Stress releases:

- Prayer, meditation and visualization— alone or in combination—are excellent tools for mental and physical health. There are myriad approaches to these disciplines. Find the ones that fit your personality and lifestyle.
- Hobbies settle the worried mind and provide a creative outlet. Artistic endeavors such as painting, potting, and photography take you away from your troubles.

▪ Sports, both spectator and participation, can reduce stress. Team sports provide camaraderie, friendship, and healthy competition. There's a sport for every fitness level, from croquet to hiking.

▪ Reading and writing—nothing takes you out of yourself more than a good book. I've always been an avid reader, but even more, I'm a writer. Almost every town has a library and writing groups. Memoir writing, poetry, fiction, and journaling are therapeutic. Writing short stories and children's books will take you from reality to fantasy. Maybe the next great novel is hidden inside you—you'll never know until you try.

▪ Movies and theater get you out of the house. Have you ever tried acting classes? Do you sing? Dance? Your heart will thank you if you try.

▪ Meaningful work will do more to heal your heart, mind, and body than any medication. If you find your day job less than meaningful, try adding work that excites and inspires you. Maybe it's a volunteer position—something you love; something you're passionate about. You know what it is.

* * *

> Kama, the Hindu god of pleasure arrived in the world with one question: "What's my job?" He knew that without purpose, life has no meaning. He also knew that creativity connects you to a higher source, one that will heal and energize.

"Dinner's ready, Blake. Will you turn that thing off?" I commanded, an edge to my voice. I hadn't seen him all day, and still he sat glued to his computer screen, working.

"One second . . . just let me finish this . . ." The usual reply.

"I said, now! You're going to go blind if you stare at that much longer."

"I know I can figure this out," he said. But then, seeing me scowling in the doorway, he reluctantly got up from his chair.

"I have no doubt," I said, "but you'll have to do it after dinner."

This scenario regularly plays out in our household. Blake is a self-employed web and multimedia designer—a business that he expands with every technological advance. The point is, he loves what he does and he's not done doing it. And I believe it's that love that has kept him alive.

Elaine—Self-Care

As primary caregiver, it's easy to give yourself away—that is, to subordinate your life totally to another's. This, I discovered, is neither effective nor healthy.

As I write this, Blake and I have been married thirty-seven years. For most of our marriage, we did everything together and had only mutual friends. It sounds ideal, but in reality such total absorption in another person can be unhealthy. As Blake's energy failed—he grew distant, removed. I felt stuck. Afraid to lose good health insurance benefits, I remained in a stressful job that under normal circumstances I would have quit. I had trouble sleeping and grew depressed. Looking for a life preserver, I found it at my local junior college—a memoir writing group. From this innocent beginning, I branched out, using writing as a vehicle to meet new people, go places, and be creative. I developed a life of my own; one that didn't conflict with my life with Blake, but added to my self-worth.

A few weeks after Blake's surgery, when he was feeling better, I waved a flyer under his nose. "Hey, look at this poetry workshop next month."

"So? I hate poetry."

"Not for you, silly. For me."

I had joined Redwood Writers, a local group whose motto is: Writers Helping Writers. The list of activities—endless: open mikes at cafés, workshops, guest speakers, theater, writing contests, and an annual anthology that showcases members' works.

"It's on a Saturday afternoon. Do you mind doing the grocery shopping that day?" I asked with a snippet of trepidation.

"No, not at all," Blake replied. "Look," he continued, "I want you to be happy . . . you were so depressed before. I felt bad—responsible."

"Really? I thought you had lost interest . . . didn't care."

"I was frightened," he said. "Each time I had an echocardiogram they told me everything looked the same, but I could feel my life slipping away. I tried not to think about it—talk about it—even to you."

"But, you should have. I felt deserted, alone. It hurt."

"I'm sorry . . . it's how I am. I can't show weakness. Have to maintain."

We sat quietly for a few seconds. Blake's eyes glistened with tears—a rare occurrence. I knew at that moment that the worst was over; we were going to be all right.

Self-Care Tips

- Maintain your routines. Whether you're caring for a parent, grandparent, child, friend or spouse, consistency alleviates fear for patient and caregiver.
- Take time for yourself. Add activities that help you relax, make friends, and feel good. You too need emotional support. It's impossible to take care of someone else if you're falling apart.
- Get away from it all. Embrace moments of solitude: take long walks in the fresh air, write, read, listen to music, pray, meditate. It's even okay to do nothing once in awhile.

- Seek hobbies as creative outlets.
- Exercise and eat right.
- Seek meaningful work, even if you don't get paid.
- Keep a pet, ideally one who dishes out regular doses of unconditional love and brightens your day.
- Seek professional help if you feel overwhelmed. You may find relief with a family counselor, therapist, or spiritual advisor such as a priest, pastor, or rabbi. Support Groups such as Mended Hearts (www.mendedhearts.org) help heart patients and their families by providing visiting services, regularly scheduled meetings, and informational seminars.
- Don't go it alone. Elicit help from friends and family members.

Journaling

I write stories, essays, poems, and books like this one. I journal in a small hardbound notebook—handwritten and free-flowing thoughts. The most private parts of me live on those pages. I show them to no one.

Each day I find a prompt—a sentence starter. Sometimes I see the words in something I read that day. Or I sit still and let the starter line come to me. It can be anything, such as:

- I love to . . .
- It's true that . . .
- Today, I should . . .
- I believe in . . .

The list is endless—find what fits your mood as you pick up a pen or pencil. Remember this is your private space—nothing is off limits. Capture feelings, especially those that may embarrass or shame you. This is a safe place to release what you don't like and reinvent yourself. Your journal doesn't lie, cheat, or steal from you. It doesn't judge or answer back. It is your true friend, because it is you.

I wrote a poem as I sat in the Intensive Care Unit listening to Blake's electronic monitors beep. I later copied it into my journal for comfort. I made an exception and shared the poem with others, and now I share it with you.

Heartfelt

Thirty-seven years
married for better or worse.
Two loving hearts
nestled in a world
of their own creation.

One heart, too big,
stopped,
faulted.
One heart, not big enough.

Lost love.
With offbeat compulsion
she sank.
Losing consciousness
he fell away.
Two hearts in need of surgery.

Could this be it? The conclusion?
What would she do without him?
Where would he go without her?

Life after death.
She prayed,
he prayed
for the same
yet different things.
Soon, a world of prayers.

God heard.
Two hearts—one repaired, one restarted.
Heartfelt recovery.

On Vacation—New Ways of Having Fun

Not long after Blake's defibrillator implant, we set off on a Hawaiian vacation. Two years later we took a dream trip to Alberta and the Canadian Rockies. We regularly flit around California and the Pacific Northwest. Seattle and Newport, Oregon, have become familiar stomping grounds. Vacations are important, not only for relaxation, but to remind us simply to have some fun.

Tips for successful travel and vacation time:

- Plan ahead and choose places that have access to emergency medical care. Check with your health-insurance carrier, and carry a list of doctors and medical-emergency providers in the area. Travel insurance is an affordable way to insure that you and your loved one are covered in an emergency.

- Reduce stress by making all travel arrangements before you leave home. Last-minute bookings can spell disaster for an exhausted heart patient. Try to drive or fly during daylight hours, and arrive at your destination prepared for an early bedtime.
- Adventure travel is no longer an option. Taking a heart patient to the Amazon rainforest is ill advised. Blake and I snorkel, kayak, and hike on our vacations, but we do it with common-sense self-restrictions. If possible, consider a group tour. Let the guide know about your charge's condition, and take it easy. Know your limitations.
- Whenever practical, prepare and eat your own food. Picnics are as much fun, if not more, than fancy restaurants or salt-laden fast-food dives. We often remark on our "table by the window" as we gaze over the mountains or ocean from our picnic blanket. Invest in some low, comfortable chairs and colorful, reusable plates and utensils to add festivity to any fresh-air breakfast, lunch, or dinner.
- When you do eat out, choose places with the freshest ingredients. Tropical islands are rich with fresh fish, fruits, and vegetables. Stick as close to your regular diet as possible, and remember not to drink too much. You'll come back from vacation slim, tan, healthy, and relaxed.
- Walk as much as possible, even in cities. When we visited Seattle, we stayed downtown, parked our car, and didn't move it until we left. Ferries, buses, and a good pair of walking shoes were all we needed to see the city and its surrounding islands. Pike's Market provided most of our meals, its vendors displaying fresh-baked breads, simply prepared fish and meats,

local fresh vegetables, and the most wonderful coffees and beers.

Peace of Mind—Blake Receives an Upgrade

Blake noticed the look of concern on the Medtronic Technician's face. "It looks like you're going to get a new ICD for Christmas," the young man said.

Blake lifted himself off the exam table. "I figured the time was getting close for a new battery."

"Well, they're not replacing batteries any longer. Instead you'll get a whole new unit. This one will be smaller and more comfortable. And while you sleep, it will communicate automatically with the modem we'll give you to place next to your bed."

"I don't understand. What will it do?"

"It notes nighttime activity and sends a report to Dr. Erickson's office. In the morning, if anything out of the ordinary has registered, the doctor's office will call to see how you feel. It's just one more safety check."

Blake laughed at the idea of a virtual connection to his doctor's office. "Well, I guess it's official. I'm the bionic man. Maybe I'll tout my electronic aid on my website—might help drum up business."

We scheduled Blake's surgery for January 2009. The procedure required anesthesia and a small incision, but was otherwise noninvasive and uneventful. We checked in at

7:30 a.m. and were home nine hours later. Blake took Tylenol for minor pain and diligently followed the usual shower routine—don't soap or wet the incision and use a clean towel each time to remain bacteria and infection-free.

The next two years were the most difficult time for us. If I could replay it, I would try to open up more, be a better communicator. Blake's failing health coincided with a natural middle-aged lull in our marriage. Even healthy people change in their fifties, and couples often find it necessary to reinvent their relationship.

Tips for keeping your family and marriage intact:

- Speak openly about your fears. If you have children, include them in these discussions. Take a positive attitude, but be honest. Pretending that nothing is wrong only adds stress.
- Be warm and polite, even when you don't feel like it. Make an extra effort to say "I love you" and mean it. A sincere "thank you" goes a long way toward soothing frayed nerves. And it goes both ways. As caregiver, be sure to express your love and appreciation for the one you support. It will uplift the spirit and heal the body.
- Take time to be alone as a couple. Escape the world long enough to love and nurture one another. Sexual relations may change, but there are many ways to physically love your partner. Try new things.
- Fight fair. All couples and families fight on occasion. The key to resolving disputes is to avoid clamming up. If you're angry, express it, and as soon as possible. Don't wallow in your anger. Be clear about the issues.

Say what's bothering you. Stick to the subject and be willing to compromise. Be specific and don't attack with insults. Listen to each other and try and find a win-win solution.

Chapter Four
The Wakeup Call

God Hits Blake Over the Head

Arriving home one evening, overloaded with work stuff, I pried open the kitchen door with my one free hand and eased inside. I slipped out of the shoulder straps of my laptop, book bag, and lunch box, and lowered it all onto the table. At first I didn't notice Blake's appearance; I saw only the blood on the floor.

"What's that? Did Jesse get hurt again?" I asked. I assumed our adopted greyhound, Jesse, had tangled with another raccoon.

"I had an episode," Blake said.

I took a step toward my husband and realized that the blood pooled at his feet had come from his head. Blood oozed from his scalp and dripped to the floor as Blake attempted to stop the flow with a kitchen towel.

"What happened? Let me see."

I dragged a chair over from the table. "Sit down." I gently pulled the blood-soaked dish towel from Blake's head, revealing a six-inch laceration.

"This looks bad. We need to go to the emergency room."

"No, I'm all right."

"No, you're not all right. How did this happen?"

"I dunno . . . I passed out."

"We're going."

After several hours and seven staples in Blake's scalp, we returned home at 10:00 p.m. In the morning, Blake called Dr. Erickson with the gory details. A remote transmission from his ICD revealed an arrhythmia serious enough to have killed him. He had gone into cardiac arrest. It was time to consider surgery.

Surgical Options

A few days later, Blake met with the office's registered nurse, Carla. "Dr. Erickson will be in shortly, but I wanted to fill you in about your condition and options," she said with nary a smile.

Blake squirmed on the edge of the exam table. "It doesn't sound like good news."

"Well, it's all how you approach it. The latest episode, as you know, was serious. The ICD saved your life. The good news is that you are otherwise in excellent health and a low risk for mitral valve surgery. More than likely the valve can be repaired and not replaced."

Carla went on to explain that the heart, as a pump, has a set of one-way flap valves. These valves regulate the blood flow to the body. Blake's valves leaked, causing his heart to overwork and consequently swell from the strain. The enlargement disrupts the electrical charge, causing arrhythmias. Blake already knew this, but he let Carla finish while he calmed his nerves with deep breaths.

"If you're in agreement that you want the surgery, I'll schedule an angiogram and a meeting with the surgeon. What do you think?" Carla gently placed her hand on Blake's shoulder.

Blake didn't hesitate. "I can't go on like this anymore. I want to get it over with. So yes, please, go ahead and schedule."

"Fine. I think that's a wise decision." She smiled and left.

As Blake waited for Dr. Erickson, he stared at the pastel art print on the wall. *Soothing color,* he thought. *I wonder where they bought it. A doctor's catalog?*

"Hey, Blake . . . you sure had a doozy. I'm glad to see you're still with us," Dr. Erickson said as he lowered himself into the chair facing his patient.

"I'm still here," Blake said in a monotone.

"Well, I consulted with the other cardiologists on the medical panel and they all agree: It's time to do the surgery. I had hoped to wait, but they're convinced, so I conceded. How do you feel about it?"

"Like I told Carla—I'm ready."

"Good. I'm going to fix you up with one of the best surgeons around. He's the senior cardiac surgeon at Pacific Coast Cardiac and Vascular Surgeons Group. Over the past twenty-five years, he's performed more than ten thousand operations focusing on valve repair and replacement. And after reviewing your last echocardiogram, I'm almost certain he'll recommend repair, which has a much shorter and easier recovery. You can have the surgery either in San Francisco or Redwood City—your choice. They're both excellent facilities."

Blake stopped at the front desk on the way out. Tia, Dr. Erickson's office manager, had Blake's information on her computer screen. "Oh. I see that you're going to see Dr. God," she said.

"What?"

"Dr. God. That's what we call Dr. Gaudiani because he works miracles. You're lucky."

"I can't say that I feel lucky, but I do feel in good hands. I'll be glad when it's all over."

"Well, I've got everything scheduled. Monday you'll have the angiogram. And you can't drive yourself . . . right?"

"No problem. My wife can take a day off work."

"Then Wednesday you'll see Dr. Gaudiani in San Francisco at one in the afternoon. That way you avoid the commute traffic."

"How soon do you think I can have the operation?"

"Hard to say. Sometime after the holidays, probably January. But you're stable now . . . so there's no rush."

Determining Factors when Considering Surgery

▪ Your doctors' recommendations. A good cardiologist welcomes a second opinion and willingly shares your information for further review.
▪ How you feel, both physically and psychologically? Has quality of life become compromised? In Blake's case, his symptoms increased to a dangerous level, making the decision easier.
▪ Success and mortality rates. Pacific Coast Cardiac and Vascular Surgeons (www.pccvs.com) provides a comprehensive, up-to-date brochure that gives the patient a full understanding of surgery results. A less than two percent mortality rate for Mitral Valve Replacement relieved our fears. In fact, the rate of death for Mitral Valve Repair is zero for patients under eighty years old. We watched a webcast procedure performed by the surgical team. Seeing the procedure done alleviated even more concerns. Over eleven years the surgical team performed 1,874 mitral-valve procedures, of which 1,192 were repairs and 682 were replacements. Ninety-seven percent of patients required no further therapy for their repaired mitral valve. If all went according to plan, Blake would be cured after surgery.
▪ Recovery time. Even though the chances of successful surgery are good, your life and the lives of those around you will be disrupted for months. Smaller incisions, now done on ninety percent of patients, reduce recovery time and are cosmetically appealing. Still, you need to weigh the financial and emotional impact that

three to six months of disability will have on your lives. Blake, self-employed, works at home, making it easier for him to ease back into work as he recovered.

▪ Cost and health insurance. How will you pay for extensive surgical and medical treatment? I have excellent health insurance through work that covers Blake. Our bills in the last six months amounted to more than $300,000, most of which were covered by insurance. If you are insured, be sure to contact your insurance company before you embark on your medical adventure. Your healthcare providers will submit your case for preapproval. This is a necessary step to insure payment of your claims. Nail down the expenses that are your responsibility. Many employers offer multiple insurance plans. Compare Health Maintenance Organizations (HMOs) with Preferred Provider Organizations (PPOs). HMOs are typically less expensive with fewer options than PPOs. Note when your employer has "open enrollment," allowing you to change plans. Double check if there are any "preexisting condition" clauses in the new plan before you switch.

▪ Individual coverage. If you're unemployed, self-employed, or retired, consider all insurance options. Each state has a public-health insurance program that provides healthcare services for the poor. The federal program, Medicare, is available to those age sixty-five and older who worked (or their spouse worked) and paid Medicare taxes for at least ten years. Many membership organizations such as AARP offer insurance coverage and Medicare supplements. In addition, check with any community and professional groups of which you're a member; they may offer group-insurance coverage. Compare available plans to find one that best meets your needs.

> Watch out for insurance scams. The Federal Trade Commission and several states have legal actions pending against fraudulent companies that offer medical discount cards. These percentage discounts often mean nothing. You need to call the provider's office and find out what charges are discounted and what's the final cost. Fraudulent health-insurance companies sell policies for coverage that is largely nonexistent. Ask for a list of providers and contact them to validate coverage. Research companies before you buy. A list of investigative resources is available in Chapter Fourteen.

Meeting Dr. Vincent Gaudiani

I took the day off work so that Blake and I could meet his surgeon together. We planned to have the procedure done at Sequoia Hospital, in Redwood City, but scheduled our meeting at the San Francisco office.

"Can you believe this traffic?" I asked Blake as we inched along Highway 101 toward the Golden Gate Bridge.

"Just our luck. We should have left sooner," he groused.

Three hours of stop-and-go traffic later, we finally made it into San Francisco. We had called ahead from the car and were told not to worry—they were behind schedule.

The four-story medical-center parking garage was packed. We finally found a spot on the top level. Already a half hour late for our appointment, we hurried down four flights of stairs and onto the crowded streets of Pacific Heights.

"Slow down," Blake pleaded. We were walking up a steep hill, and he was lagging behind, panting.

"Oh, sorry. I don't like it here . . . too congested."

"Well I'm congested too, remember? You'll give me another heart attack."

I slowed my pace, realizing that I felt closed in by the stressful day. Slow down and relax, I told myself. "I'm sorry, Blake. Are you okay? I didn't realize I was pushing so hard. Here, give me your hand."

"I'm fine. Let's just get there." But he took my hand.

The receptionist looked up as we entered and approached her desk. "Hi. Your name?"

"Blake. Blake Webster. We're a little late . . . got stuck in traffic."

"No worries. Dr. Gaudiani is running late, too. He had an extra surgery this morning. He'll be here shortly . . . have a seat."

We fell into the waiting-room seats, breathing deeply and trying to relax. The room was crowded with patients. The change in scheduling had pushed everyone's appointments back an hour or two. In one corner, an Asian couple chatted in Chinese. Nearby, a stocky, older man and his plump wife shifted nervously in their chairs. People paced between the restroom and the water cooler. Others flipped through piles of dog-eared magazines while periodically glancing at the door, then their watches.

Two fit-looking men in green surgical scrubs appeared in the doorway. Both sported dark tans—I pictured them on the golf course. They disappeared into their offices, and soon the receptionist began to call patients' names. The room cleared, leaving only Blake and me. Finally:

"Mr. Webster? The doctor will see you now."

As we stood, Dr. Gaudiani appeared at the door, extended his hand to Blake, then turned to me. I held out my hand and said, "I'm Elaine—Blake's wife."

He grazed my open palm with his. "C'mon in. Have a seat." He looked beat.

The spacious office had a high ceiling and expensive furnishings. We lowered into chairs around a small oval table. I pulled out Blake's medical binder, prepared to answer questions. I felt uncomfortable, out of place, but told myself to relax and breathe. The doctor opened Blake's medical file.

"First, I want you to know that you're special. We rarely see anyone who has had cardiac arrest. You'd be dead without that ICD in your chest."

"So I've been told."

"When did you last have the unit replaced?"

I opened the binder and found the right page. Blake said, "January 2009."

As a caregiver, it's hard to get used to taking a backseat to the patient. Most healthcare professionals will allow you access to meetings and examinations, but expect you to be only a spectator. The conversation is between doctor and patient. So it helps to prepare your questions ahead and let the patient ask them. You can take an active role by taking notes.

Dr. Gaudiani, focused on Blake, picked up a plastic heart. On the sidelines, I relaxed my shoulders and concentrated on deep breathing from my diaphragm—an anxiety-relieving technique.

The doctor smiled weakly and leaned back in his chair. It had obviously been a long day for him; I tried to send good thoughts his way.

"So, this is the problem with your heart," he said, brandishing his plastic replica. "Each time it beats, it pumps blood to the rest of your body. This valve, here, is the mitral valve and yours is flapping instead of opening and closing, causing blood to leak back into the lungs. It's why you're so congested. A normal heart pumps enough blood each day to fill a hot tub. You'd be lucky to fill it a quarter of the way. But we're going to fix that."

"And it's enlarged too, isn't it?" Blake asked.

Dr. Gaudiani rolled up the right sleeve of his green surgical scrubs, exposing a muscular bicep. I took another deep breath—this time out of admiration. He flexed his arm and pointed at his bulging muscle.

"It's like this: you work a muscle and it gets larger. In the arm, that's a good thing. For the heart, it's not. An enlarged heart misaligns the normal electrical path that makes it beat. When the path is disrupted, the heart vibrates instead of pulsing. The arrhythmia without a defibrillation shock to return the natural heart rhythm is what kills you."

"Dr. Erickson said to ask you about something called the Maze operation," Blake said.

The doctor hesitated. "Well, I don't think that will help you. It works well for Atrial Fibrillation, but you have Ventricular Fibrillation. Maze is a procedure where we make tiny cuts around the heart, then sew them up so as to redirect the electrical current. Again, I don't think it's warranted in your case."

"So, Dr. Erickson thinks you'll be able to repair the valve?"

"Oh, it's definitely a repair job. You'll be as good as new. I've done thousands of these procedures, and no one under eighty years old has ever died on me."

"That's what I heard. How soon can I have it done?"

"Sometime after the holidays. Or you could wait awhile, if you want. You're stabilized now—no urgency."

"No, I want to do it as soon as possible. I want to get it over with and get back to normal. This passing-out thing really freaked me out."

"Okay. Talk to Jane up front. You'll need someone home with you for at least a week afterwards."

"I plan to take two weeks off from work," I butted in. "I'm fortunate to have enough leave time."

"Good, then it's set. We'll do it here at the hospital, and afterward we have a place you can stay. It's down the hill, but we run a shuttle . . ."

"I hoped we could go to Redwood City," I said, cutting the doctor off in midsentence. "The city's so crowded and scary for me to get around—"

"Oh, sure. Makes no difference." With that, he got up and headed for the door.

Blake and I gathered up our belongings and walked out to the reception desk. It had been a long day for the office staff, too. A weary Jane gave us the first available date—January 14.

"I'll mail you more information," she said. "If you have any further questions, just call the Redwood City office. Do you want to stay at the hostel? It's free to families, on a first-come, first-serve basis."

"I hoped to find a moderately priced motel," I answered.

"I'll send you a list that gives discounts for hospital patients and their families."

* * * *

The next few weeks moved at a snail's pace. Blake's energy waned, and the holidays passed with little joviality and increased anxiety for us both. Blake, while working in his office, had another episode a week before the scheduled surgery. He called Dr. Erickson's office and spoke with Carla.

"I almost fainted again," he said weakly.

"Oh, Blake, I'm sorry," Carla said in her most comforting voice. "I know you don't want to hear this, but just hang in there. Everything's set. Your ICD is there to keep you alive, and surgery is in place. You'll make it . . . try and relax."

I began to cross off the days on the calendar. Seven more days to go.

Chapter Five
Ready and Set

Picking the Best—Sequoia Hospital in Redwood City

Long before we chose Dr. Gaudiani and his surgical team, we'd heard of Sequoia Hospital in Redwood City. One Friday afternoon, as I lingered outside the Community Church in Sebastopol, I chatted with members of my memoir-writing group.

"So, Elaine, how's Blake?" Chuck asked. He knew that a week earlier I'd found my husband wobbling and bleeding in the kitchen.

"Well, it appears we're looking at surgery. We've put it off for twelve years, but the last episode told us it's time," I said.

I pulled my jacket collar up to block the wind as Steve, our instructor, approached. He gave me a quick hug and I thought how he looked more like a trailblazer than a writing teacher. The cold front had forced him to trade in hiking shorts for jeans—the trail shoes were a constant.

"Sure is cold out here today," he said with chattering teeth. "How's Blake?"

I repeated what I'd said about the operation, and barely got the words out when Chuck put in, "Where are you having the surgery done?"

"We're meeting with a surgeon that operates at both Sequoia Hospital in Redwood City and in San Francisco."

"Oh, you want to go to Redwood City . . . yes . . . definitely Redwood City," Chuck insisted.

"Why, what's the difference?" I asked.

"I have several friends who had their heart surgeries there. People travel from all over the world to Sequoia Hospital because of its high success rate. They attract some of the best doctors, surgeons, and healthcare professionals in the world. The facility has state-of-the-art technology and friendly staff. You'll be in good hands."

I glanced around as my classmates arrived—some alone, others in groups of twos and threes. Despite the chill, they lingered outside, chattering and laughing. The Santa Rosa Junior College catalog lists the memoir class in its Older Adults program, but there is no age minimum and students range in age from fifty to ninety-something. Some overcome disabilities to get here. Sylvia has a new fancy power wheelchair; Thelma Jean, still sharp of mind in her seventies, walks several blocks with the help of leg braces and crutches. Jeremy, a survivor of brain surgery, shuffles when he walks but writes brilliantly.

Jeremy and I usually arrive first, and I look forward to our conversations after a long work week. His gentle manner calms me and his humor cheers me. He offers simple advice with great insights.

"You seem so calm about Blake's surgery," he said.

"I'm scared inside, but there's no point in talking much about it. People don't want to hear your troubles. Even here, I've been cut off mid-sentence, and it hurts. Feeling vulnerable, I find myself keeping to myself more and more."

"Except for your writing," Jeremy said. "We all love your writing."

"Thanks, but I've been trying some new styles and I don't think they're going over too well. I guess I'm going through an insecure phase. At first I felt empowered by my writing, now I feel diminished."

"Believe me, I know how you feel. Surgeries, doctors and hospitals affect you more than you think. The disruption of daily life, the worry, the unknown . . . it's hard. You'll be all right . . . you'll see. And you're writing will be better for the experience."

Steve looked at his watch, then at the oak door. "Okay guys and girls, it's time."

Younger students help their elderly friends get settled in the circle, all the while chatting away about books, movies, concerts, theater, and current writing projects. Ensconced among the cushions of one of the couches, I listen to tales of love, loss, and adventure, and reflect on the frailty of life. I think of Blake, his damaged heart, and all that blood. *What if he died? What would I do without him? . . . Don't think about that. Try to relax—you're among friends here. Look at what others have overcome. Thelma Jean had a stroke. Sylvia recently lost her husband of fifty years. We can do this . . .*

A Day of Caring

A young woman with a kind smile welcomed us to America's Best Inn, on El Camino Real in Redwood City. The strong smell of curry reminded me I was hungry.

"We have a reservation and a special rate," Blake offered. "I'm going into surgery tomorrow, and Sequoia Hospital said you'd be flexible about checkout times. We don't know how many days it will be."

The woman straightened her sari and spoke in an Indian accent. "No worries. We understand. Hospital patients and their families stay here often. We can leave your bill open as long as you pay for two nights ahead. Then we'll settle up at the end."

Blake pulled his reading glasses from his pocket, maneuvered them on, and peered at the registration card. "Could you get the license-plate number off the car?" he said to the air as he began to write. Knowing the words were meant for me, I went out to the parking lot with pen and scratch paper—a ritual repeated every time we check into a motel.

With no elevator available, Blake lugged our suitcase up the single flight of stairs, stopping every few seconds to catch his breath. I followed with two laptop computers. I glanced at the pool, then at the shabby-looking apartments next door. Gym equipment, bicycles, plastic chairs and tables filled the balconies. A few of the windows had faded bed sheets as curtains.

I swiped the key card and pushed open the door. Flecks of Mylar confetti dotted the brown carpet. "Looks like someone had a birthday party in here—they need a stronger vacuum cleaner," I said.

While Blake returned to the car for a second load, I pulled open the drapes and surveyed our temporary home. The room was clean, but a bit shabby. Glad to see a writing desk, I set the computer cases on it and poked around. A TV and DVD player hid behind the closed doors of an armoire with more than a few dings. An archway divided the bathroom/kitchen area from the rest of the room. Unpainted caulking filled the biggest holes in the counter-top. The small refrigerator, coffee pot, and microwave would come in handy. The Whole Foods store across the street would provide the ingredients for simple meals.

"Not too bad, eh?" Blake set a bag of kitchen essentials on the counter.

"It's fine," I replied, putting my arms around Blake's waist. "I don't plan to spend much time here anyway. I'll be with you at the hospital. It's just a place to sleep . . . what time's our appointment at the hospital?"

"Nine o'clock—we need to go now."

* * *

The admittance clerk verified Blake's personal information and took a photocopy of the insurance card. I filled out a form that listed people from whom Blake would accept phone calls. I wanted to screen Blake's calls—I wrote "none."

"Do you have a co-pay?" the young, brown-haired woman asked as she pulled our information up on her computer screen.

"I think so, but I'm not sure what it is," I answered.

"Well, let's not worry about that now. It looks like you have excellent coverage. They want us to get the co-pays up front, but I prefer to wait. I hate taking money from people before we even know what's owed. You can mail a payment later after we bill you."

"Sounds good to me," I said.

Second stop—the admittance interview, Nurse Angela's office. She gestured for us to sit, then produced a pile of forms for us to complete and sign.

"This paperwork never ends," she said. "By the time we're done, we'll know more about you than you do. Now where's that other form? Hold on a second, I'll be right back. I need to make some more copies."

With barely enough room for two chairs, I scooted aside to let the nurse by, all the time feeling on edge and out of place. Medical etiquette required that Angela speak directly to the patient, but it always makes me feel like an extra in a movie.

Angela returned. "Okay, I think we're set. First I need you to sign this permission for an HIV test, a standard requirement. Then I'll take some blood. We also take a nasal swab to check for MRSA (methicillin resistant staphylococcus), a serious bacterial infection that is highly resistant to some antibiotics. You may have heard about some recent hospital outbreaks. The symptoms, which include rashes and skin infection, can be severe in patients with compromised health. But don't worry, we haven't had a problem here because of good prescreening."

Angela completed the two tests and attached Blake's identification wrist bands. "Now don't let anyone do anything to you or administer any drugs without first checking these bands and asking your name and birthdate. It will become a ritual you'll soon tire of, but it prevents mistakes."

Blake signed more paperwork that documented what operation was to be performed and by which surgeon.

"Here's some preoperative information," Angela said as she passed Blake two sheets of paper. One sheet had a line drawing of a naked man, without genitalia. His name—Surgery Sam. Sam's chest was highlighted in yellow. Angela handed Blake a box of antiseptic wipes and explained how to use them. The morning before surgery he would thoroughly clean all areas of his body where bacteria congregate. The second set of wipes was to be used on the area noted on Surgery Sam. At the hospital, before surgery, Blake would be shaved and scrubbed again. Angela also gave Blake an antiseptic mouthwash of Chlorhexidine Gluconate, to reduce the risk of catching a cold virus. She then administered a standard EKG (electrocardiography) to record Blake's heart rhythms, and we were done.

"All right, now take the elevator to the second floor medical lab for some more blood work. Give them this folder and they'll know what to do. Any questions?"

"No, I think we've got it," Blake said, taking the folder.

Blake stared straight ahead as I pushed the elevator button.

"You okay?" I asked him.

He just shrugged.

The lab took Blake right away, and I found an empty seat in front of the television screen, tuned to CNN. Recoiling from the relentless assault of bad news, I picked up the local free entertainment newspaper. Unable to focus, I stared at its pages without reading a word. I wanted to be somewhere else, anywhere else.

Finally after a half hour, Blake emerged from the medical testing lab. He looked pale.

"That was quick," I said, mustering a smile.

"I'm surprised I have any blood left. I counted ten vials of blood by the time they were finished," he said, again without humor. I was worried.

We had an hour to kill before traipsing up the hill to the Pacific Coast Cardiac and Vascular Surgeons (PCCVS) office. To orient ourselves, we took a self-guided tour of the hospital. Around every corner, friendly staff smiled and offered directions. We located our morning check-in point—the Short Stay Unit.

"So, I think we've got it together to this point," I said to Blake. "How do you feel?"

"Poked and prodded like a piece of meat."

I took his hand and held it as we climbed the hill to the PCCVS office. We were both out of breath as we entered the second-floor suite of offices. A PCCVS staffer greeted us at the reception window. Given more forms to fill out, we sank into an oversized sofa and I handed Blake his glasses.

"So much for a paperless society," Blake said as he started scribbling. "All these forms ask the same questions."

While Blake wrote, I leaned my head back and closed my eyes until a voice interrupted my mini-nap. "Is this your first heart surgery?" I opened my eyes and saw a middle-aged woman with a clipboard sitting across from us. "I'm Pat, a volunteer from *The Mended Hearts*. We're a nation-wide heart-patient support organization. Would you like to talk?"

Dubious and tired, I managed a weak smile. Blake still had his head buried in paperwork. Pat continued,

“Starting as a teenager, I’ve had three valve-replacement surgeries.”

I didn’t like hearing that. “Three? How come three?”

“Forty years ago, heart surgery was nothing like it is today. My first surgery almost killed me and I spent two weeks in the hospital, with many months of recovery. The pig valve lasted ten years, then it had to be replaced. I pilot glider planes for fun, so I couldn’t risk passing out from an arrhythmia during flight. The second surgery was easier and my third one, last year, went even better.”

Blake looked up. “How long did it take for you to recover that last time?”

“I was in the hospital for three days after surgery. Then I guess it took about four months before I felt okay and two more months until I was fully recovered—six months total. But then each of my surgeries was a new replacement. If you have a repair you’ll feel better sooner.”

“How about the actual surgery? Blake asked. “We watched a webcast and it looked fairly routine.”

“Let’s just say, you’re fortunate to have Dr. Gaudiani. He gets in, gets the job done, and gets out. The longer you’re on heart-lung bypass, the more traumatized your body and the longer the recovery. This surgical team is world-renown for its expertise and efficiency. They’ve worked together for years, functioning as a well-oiled machine.”

Pat handed me her clipboard and I wrote down our contact information. The Santa Rosa chapter of *The Mended Hearts* would be in touch. Before she left, Pat handed me a colorful packet containing pages of information and a copy of *Heartbeat* magazine. One of the articles was titled "Then & Now: The past 20 years have seen huge advances in cardiac care."

Slipping the magazine into my briefcase for a later read, I thought, *I like the sound of that.*

* * *

"Blake?" A young male technician emerged from a side corridor.

"That's me," Blake said with no enthusiasm.

"C'mon in and we'll get you started. First I'll do an EKG, then Wilson, one of our physician assistants, will finish your final exam before surgery."

"I'll wait here," I said, but no one appeared to hear me. Blake disappeared with the technician and I returned to my nap.

* * *

Four p.m. found us back in our motel room. I put away groceries, while Blake set up connections for the computers. The wi-fi worked well. While Blake checked his messages, I sent out the first of many group emails.

Hi all,

Here's the first APB.

We just finished our preliminary meet-and-greets with hospital admissions, with Mended Hearts (a heart patient advocacy nonprofit), and with Dr. Gaudiani's (surgeon) office. Blake's been poked and prodded for the last time before surgery, and we have a pretty good idea of what to expect. What makes Blake different (among other things) is that he went into cardiac arrest the night he hit his head and even though he's on an anti-arrhythmia drug, he had another episode last Wednesday. Still, optimism is high and we're assured that we are in the best of care. Even the health advocate told us that Dr. Gaudiani and his team are considered some of the best in the world and international patients are common.

Are we nervous? You bet. The ICU will be the most stressful. Blake will be "tubed up" on a respirator and chest tubes. They will allow me access as much as they can, but at first probably only 10–15 minutes at a time. He may be in intensive care from one to two days. Then he'll be moved to a room for another three to four days. On the way home (two-hour drive) we'll need to stop several times for him to stretch his legs to prevent clots. The key to everything is to keep him moving as much as possible and out of pain. The good news is that they are planning a relatively small incision.

Apparently, there's an infamous day three, when the body decides to become majorly pissed off about its plight and patients get angry and sometimes verbally abusive. I can't see it for Blake, but I've been forewarned to not take anything he says personally at that time. Yikes!

Anyway, we're back in our room, both on our computers. Blake's fixing a client's website which at least gets his mind off stuff. I'm messing around with you guys. The motel is walking distance to Whole Foods, so good food is easily obtained at a reasonable price. We're scheduled for 8:00 a.m. surgery and will check in at 6:00. The hospital has wi-fi throughout, so I'll send out email updates as the news breaks.

If anything bad happens, I'll call; otherwise email is less stressful for me. Feel free to email me anytime.

Love,
Elaine

We were a somber pair that night. The impending surgery was like a ghost, haunting our room. In contrast to our usual pattern of chatting about our days, we said little. Fear was our constant companion. Time crawled, filled with a light dinner salad, bad television, and a glass of Port wine to make us sleepy. We crawled into bed at nine-thirty, but neither of us fell asleep.

I hugged Blake close to me. "It's going to be all right, you know."

"I know. I feel like I'm in the Twilight Zone, where nothing is real. I want to be on the other side of this surgery. I want to be home, in my own bed. I want to be well."

"We're on this adventure together, just remember that. I'll be close the entire time. We'll make it through . . . we'll make it through."

Chapter Six
Surgery Day

Short Stay Unit: Answered Prayers

We reported early Friday morning, January 14, 2011, to the Short Stay Unit. They were expecting us.

"Blake, come this way and we'll get you prepped," the nurse said. "Elaine, you can take a seat over there. We'll come get you when he's done, and you can sit with him until it's time to go in."

I sat and glanced awkwardly at the fidgety man sitting across from me: mid-thirties, medium build, blank stare. Stay away, my inner voice said.

I opened my laptop to test out the hospital's wi-fi connection.

Internet Voucher

In order to keep you connected during your time here, Catholic Healthcare West and its affiliate healthcare providers are happy to provide our patients and guests free wireless Internet connectivity. Follow the instructions below to create your personal Internet account.

Distracted, I read that opening four times before it registered.

"William? Bill?" the nurse called.

"Here," the man across from me said.

"Did someone come with you?" asked the nurse.

"No, I'm here alone."

"Well, we can't let you drive after the procedure."

"I'll call a cab."

"Okay, then . . . let's get started."

Alone—that barren word. I felt for this stranger. Was there no one to call? No one to come? That could be me if something happened to Blake. I stared at the CHW guest login page. I had to choose a Username and Password, but I couldn't muster the energy. I shut down the computer and sat staring at the wall. A few minutes later the nurse called my name.

"Mrs. Webster, you can go back now. Blake's in Bay Three."

I thought of one of Blake's and my favorite Steve Goodman albums, *Jessie's Jig*, and the song, "Door Number Three."

They found us in the lost and found, love is blind but now I see
That my whole world lies waiting behind door number three
Yes, my whole world lies waiting behind door number three

I forced a smile and pulled the curtain aside, revealing a hospital-gowned husband propped up on a stretcher. I took his hand.

"Well here we are . . . what's next?"

"They told me that the surgical nurse and anesthesiologist would be in to talk to us in awhile." Blake smiled, but I could see his, too, was forced. I sat on the steel chair to his right. The patient on the other side of the curtain was giving his nurse a hard time.

"What medications do you take," the nurse asked.

"Don't you have all that in the computer? You're always asking me the same questions, and I can't remember the answers," he barked.

"Things change and we have to double-check each time. I'll go down a list and you can tell me what sounds familiar," she said patiently.

Blake and I rolled our eyes in unison. I had our medical binder ready when Dr. Gaudiani's surgical nurse, Sylvia, came in to "answer all our questions." First, she had some questions of her own—the usual ones regarding medications, overall health, dizziness, etc. After she updated Blake's responses in the computer, Sylvia extended a warm hand to us both. Her sincere, reassuring smile unknotted my stomach and I began to relax. She would be back in about fifteen minutes to take Blake to the Operating Room.

The next visitor was the anesthesiologist, an Asian man with an unpronounceable name. We surmised through his thick Chinese accent that he had worked with Dr. Gaudiani's team for years. He also said I didn't need to wait at the hospital during the surgery—someone would call me at the motel.

"But Sylvia just told us that Dr. Gaudiani would come see me personally after the operation to let me know how it went," I said.

"You can wait if you want . . . but it's not necessary," he said.

"For me it's necessary."

"Okay, do whatever you want," he said dismissively. He flipped through his folder, occasionally asking a question about Blake's condition (which Blake answered once we understood his words), then he abruptly turned and left.

"I'm not leaving you," I said, taking Blake's hand. Just then Sylvia came in to wheel Blake to surgery. Wanting to be certain that I should wait at the hospital while Blake was in surgery, I looked at her and said, "There's a waiting room nearby?"

"Yes, of course . . . down the hall."

I trailed along behind as she rolled my husband to the door. This was where we said goodbye.

"Give him a kiss," Sylvia said. "Next time you meet, this will all be over and he'll be in ICU."

I kissed Blake, squeezed his hand, and a second later they were gone.

Hours later, back at the motel room, I wrote my second APB email:

Dear Friends and Family,

This morning around 8:00, I gave Blake a kiss and watched as the surgical nurse wheeled him through swinging doors to the operating room. The moment I had anxiously awaited—now here—no way to turn back now. I looked at my feet and commanded them to move along the corridor to the ICU waiting room—it would be awhile.

I settled into a chair near an electrical socket and plugged in my laptop. The same technology that Blake adores, allows me to bring all of you with me on this medical adventure—nothing short of a miracle, really. Not too many years ago, I would have been widowed too young. Today, I wait as one of the best cardiovascular surgeons in the world performs what he considers a routine operation. Sequoia Hospital in Redwood City is a top-rated facility that prepares and informs both patient and family for the day and the weeks to come. By the end of yesterday, we had a two-inch-thick file and four-inch binder to convince us that all would be fine. Another transition in our lives completed, with many more years as "partners in crime" to come.

I struck up a conversation with Karen and her mother, Sandy, in the waiting room. They had traveled from Fresno, where Blake was born, to see Dr. Gaudiani. Sandy's husband, now 72, was being evaluated for a third heart surgery. In spite of the uncertain future, they laughed at my jokes (bad as they were) and offered me a myriad of snacks snuggled in a canvas tote. We talked about our friends and families and how fortunate we are and how much we have to be thankful for. Sandy wore a laminated pin that said, "God provides and protects." Her gold cross hung proudly across her chest. I clasped the turquoise necklace Blake bought me a few birthdays ago. It's a Tibetan design, with a picture of the Dalai Lama inside, a large Sanskrit OM design on its face. Those two religious symbols felt right hanging side by side as two wives hugged and exchanged blessings.

About noon, I heard Dr. Gaudiani's booming voice echo the hall: "Websters? Where are the Websters?"

"I'm here," I said as I rose and followed the voice.

Vincent Gaudiani doesn't walk, he bounces. When finally he stopped and faced me, he poked my upper chest. "We did the smallest possible incision, from here to about here." He laughed. "And it went well, he's fine . . . you can see him in about thirty minutes. Just pick up the ICU phone, give your name, and they'll let you in. Well, gotta go . . . see ya in a month for a follow up." And he was gone, his voice trailing off down the hall.

I thought I might be able to stay at Blake's bedside until he awoke, but the hustle and bustle of ICU only had me in the way. I stayed a few minutes, gazing at my sleeping spouse, then left for some lunch and downtime. So, after I finish this email to you, I'm off to see if the patient's awake. But before I do, I want to thank you all for your support, prayers, and good thoughts. We couldn't have done it without you.

Elaine

Intensive Care Unit

At three p.m. I picked up the wall phone outside the door of the ICU. The informational flyer stated that no visitors were allowed between two and four p.m. I hoped they'd make an exception.

"Hello?" a female voice answered.

"This is Elaine Webster, Blake Webster's wife. Can I come in?"

"Hold on, I'll check with his nurse."

A few minutes later, a young woman in hospital garb appeared. "I'm Barbara, Blake's nurse . . . c'mon in. He's in unit ten, on the left."

Nervous, I approached Blake's bed. He'd been asleep when I left, with the respirator tubing in place. Now he was untethered and awake, if you want to call it that.

"Hi, sweetie." I leaned over and kissed him on the forehead.

He looked at me, as though through a heavy ground fog. "Oh, hi."

A nurse entered. I moved aside to give her access to the computer. "So, how's he doing?" I asked.

"Good. His potassium's low, though. I'll have to ask the doctor if we should give a supplement. My guess is, we'll want to wait for now, but I'll check."

"Can I have water? I'm so thirsty," Blake whispered.

I spied a plastic glass of ice on the tray table and reached for it. The nurse stopped me with a warning. "I need you to ask before you do or give him anything. He can't have liquids until the anesthesia wears off. He'll only throw it up. He's already had one ice cube—"

"Just one more?" Blake asked weakly.

"One more, but that's it. We don't want you vomiting again."

"Again?" I asked, as the nurse turned to leave.

"Yeah," Blake answered. "She left a glass of water for me . . . thought it was okay to drink . . . made me throw up . . . still nauseous . . . pain pills make it worse . . . checking if I can take something else."

"Here, let me comb your hair and mustache. There's sticky stuff in it."

I pulled a comb from my purse and gently loosened the goop from the affected areas—leftover glue from the tape that had held the respirator in place. Blake's eyes looked like milk glass, but his skin color was good. I had mentally prepared myself for the worst; he looked better than I'd expected.

"Sweetie, you don't look bad at all. Are you comfortable? Can I do anything?"

"Can you pull the covers over my feet more? They're cold."

I adjusted Blake's blankets and surveyed the room. I now understood why the *Welcome to the Intensive Care Unit* brochure called it "a busy, noisy and unfamiliar place." Curtained bays lined the walls of the rectangular room. Computer work stations filled most of the remaining floor space, along with a medication dispensary. As I watched, a nurse entered a security code to gain access to drawers of pills and potions under the watchful eye of the head nurse. No mistakes—no missing medications.

An ear-splitting alarm sounded. A cart with a portable defibrillator was rolled to a nearby bedside. A nurse shouted, "Wake up!—open your eyes!—wake up!" She clapped her hands near the man's face. They placed the defibrillator paddles on his chest, and someone called, "Clear!" The man's body jumped, and the monitor beeped back to life.

The scene before me played out like a television hospital drama, a combination of soap opera and real life. This windowless room was a reflection of a class society. At the bottom, the invisible janitorial staff moved silently through the unit. I watched as a stocky middle-aged woman set up signs,"Caution: Wet Floor," then set about mopping. Nurses and clerical staff hustled about, doing most of the work. Doctors, in expensive suits and sweaters, stood out as the elite.

“Oh, look at you today, all dressed in black—very chic,” a handsome male doctor in an expensive Irish knit sweater remarked to an impeccably attired female doctor.

“Well, I know how you like ladies of the night,” she flirted back, her eyes never leaving her computer screen.

As a government worker, I knew that most employee manuals forbade workplace flirtation, lest it spill over into sexual harassment. Here, flirting seemed to be part of the culture. No doubt such playful remarks made long shifts go faster and lightened moods. However briefly, it took their minds off illness and death.

A few desks down, two nurses—one man, one woman—bantered about Charlie Sheen and the previous night’s *Two and a Half Men* episode.

“That show’s just not believable. No one could drink that much and keep it up,” the woman remarked.

“Oh I could,” the man said. “Want to find out some night after work?”

“With you? No way . . . besides, the med dispenser is out of Viagra.”

“How do you know? Did you empty it for that loser you went out with last week?”

“What are you two doing? Break’s over—get started on rounds—pronto!” the head nurse barked. Her tone invited no argument. Apparently mid-thirties, she wore a tight t-shirt that showcased her well-defined biceps. Her stetho-scope dangled between sizeable bosoms. Her subordi-nates jumped to work.

With nothing else fun to watch, I was glad to see a doctor approach with Blake's nurse in tow. They hovered over Blake's bed. "I'm Dr. Kardon. Dr. Gaudiani asked me to check on you. How are you feeling?"

"I'm thirsty, but every time I take a sip of water, I throw up."

"That's normal. But I'll change your pain med to Oxycodon, which is easier on the stomach."

The doctor looked at the heart monitor and said to the air, "You have A-Fib . . . you'll need to take Coumadin."

"Coumadin? What's that?" I asked.

"Blood thinner."

"This is the first we heard of it. Are there side effects?"

"Change of lifestyle," he answered cryptically and walked away, leaving the nurse to finish up with Blake.

I looked at the nurse, hoping my look of quizzical concern would prompt her to explain. She turned away and began typing at the computer.

A moment later, she glanced at Dr. Kardon, who had his back to us at the nurse's station, and said, "Don't worry, it'll all be explained later."

The doctor turned and stared. "What are you telling them?"

"Just what you said, that Blake will need Coumadin."

* * *

"You need to leave now." It was another of Blake's nurses, speaking in what sounded like a Polish or Czech accent. "It's six-thirty—time to go."

"But he's still nauseous from the potassium supplement you gave him. Can't I stay longer?"

Her face softened. "Oh, I feel bad about that. Low potassium levels contribute to A-fib, but if I'd known he had such a sensitivity I'd have waited. I'm afraid I made him feel worse."

"What's this A-fib you and Dr. Kardon keep mentioning?" I asked.

"After heart surgery about sixty percent of patients have atrial fibrillation. It's not as serious as ventricular fibrillation, but because the upper chambers of the heart quiver, it's a potential site for blood clots to form. If a clot breaks free, Blake could have a stroke. It's why Dr. Kardon wants him on Coumadin—to thin the blood, prevent clots and a potential stroke."

The word stroke made me even more reluctant to leave Blake's side. What if something happened and I wasn't here? "Are you sure I can't stay longer?"

"I'd let you if I could, but it's time for a shift change and you'll be in the way. Don't worry, we'll take good care of him. Plus you look beat. Have you eaten anything today?"

"A few snacks . . . I guess I should get some dinner." I leaned over Blake, who had dozed off. Not wanting to wake him, I kissed the top of his head, brushed stray strands of hair from his face, and grabbed my purse.

* * * *

Whole Foods market was packed with dinnertime shoppers. I wandered in circles for fifteen minutes trying to decide what to eat—nothing appealed. Wandering down the canned soup aisle, I realized I hadn't packed a can opener. I found the kitchen gadget section—can openers were fifteen dollars. I put the soup back and went to the salad bar and deli section. I finally settled on a whole rotisserie chicken, salad, and dinner rolls. I'd be hungry later, and I could stash the leftovers in the refrigerator for tomorrow.

It was a short walk across the street to the motel. In the lobby, I watched several young men, well-dressed women hanging on their arms, enter and head upstairs. For some reason, the words "escort service" leaped to mind. Regardless, they'll soon be having more fun than I will. I thought about the confetti stuck to the carpet in my room and wished I had a more festive reason for staying there.

I traipsed up the stairs, to Room 214. Once inside, I set the bag of groceries on the counter and unpacked my laptop computer. As it booted up, I opened a bottle of Port and filled a wine glass. I got a plate, piled it with food, and settled in front of the computer. Catching a glimpse of my reflection in the wall mirror, I thought, Better wash my hair tonight. I took a bite of chicken, wiped off my fingers, and hit the keyboard.

To my delight, my email box was brimming with kind words:

> Been thinking about you and Blake . . .often. Sending good vibes, thoughts and hopes for courage, serenity and happy outcomes.
>
> I'm here if you need me. If you need me to come to Redwood City. My cell, it's always on.
>
> Love, Katie

> I'm right there with you, too. Holding my breath, then releasing slow and steady, and remembering to remind you through the love channel—to deep breathe. Again, call anytime if you need anything, day or night.
>
> Big love, Rose

Give Blake a peck on the cheek from me . . . or maybe a chuck on the chin, and the peck from you.

Steve

Yeah!!!

Debbie

Elaine – I am so relieved! Thank you for the email. I look forward to many more years of partnership in crime too! Give my best to Blake, and please take care of yourself.

Love, Mark

This has seriously cheered me up.

Tell him to take care, and we look forward to hearing more good news and also to talking to Blake when he gets back into the swing of things.

Take Care

All of the Morgans in Northern Ireland

Yea!! I was sure it was going to go well but so glad to hear it confirmed. Thanks for the update. I hope the coming week isn't too bad. Though I bet Blake is going to be so glad to get this behind him that it will help with the discomfort.

Warmly, Teri

Chapter Seven
Two Days and Counting

Day Two in ICU

Next morning I was surprised to find the steel doors to the ICU propped open. I looked left and right before giving myself permission to enter unannounced. I maneuvered though the maze of computer stations and made a beeline to Blake's bedside.

"What time is it?" Blake asked. "I wondered where you were."

"Ten o'clock. The rules say no visitors before ten. How ya feeling?"

The words tumbled out. "My stomach's upset again. Every time they give me a pain pill, I get sick. And they keep switching nurses on me. I can't remember the name of the medication Dr. Kardon prescribed, and they keep giving me the one that makes me sick. I hate throwing up. I wish you could get here earlier. I can't remember anything. I need someone to keep track of what they give me."

"Is there a problem?" I flinched at the sound of the nurse's voice behind me.

I took a step back and bumped the rolling computer stand, almost knocking it over. I steadied it and myself, then asked the young blond nurse about the nausea.

"He says he's still nauseous—is that normal? The doctor said yesterday that he should have Oxycodone for pain. The other medication makes him sick, but it seems that's what he keeps getting."

"I didn't get those instructions," she replied. "Let me look . . ."

As the nurse flipped through Blake's chart, I adjusted his pillows.

"Oh, I see it now. Okay, we'll give that the next go-round. Now it's time to try a walk."

"A walk already?" Blake had been on the operating table only 24 hours ago.

"The sooner the better. Let me show you how to get him up. We'll only go a short way, but we need to get things moving."

I looked in Blake's eyes and wondered how long it would be before they sparkled again. His wrinkled forehead and dull expression reflected exhaustion and fear. I asked him if he was in pain and he said no, but he didn't want to move. The insistent nurse lowered the bed, and helped swing his legs around to the side as he struggled to lift his torso. Once his feet were firmly planted on the floor, she pulled him into her arms and they stood up together.

"There. How does that feel?" she asked.

"Okay, I think," Blake mumbled.

"Do you think you can take a few steps?"

"I think so."

I stepped aside and watched as patient and nurse shuffled away. I wanted to be helpful in some way. Instead, I stood awkwardly behind. Oh, to be home and have this over. I watched as the couple, joined like Siamese twins, reached the end of the curtained bays and turned back.

Oblivious to the rolling food cart approaching from behind, I jumped at the sound of its squeaky wheels. It was pushed by an elderly woman in street clothes.

The woman smiled. "Relax. I know this is a lot to take in, but believe me, it will be all right . . . you couldn't be in better hands. I'll set lunch over here on the counter. It looks like your wanderer has returned."

The nurse helped Blake ease into a chair. After checking the monitors and making entries in the computer, she left to continue her rounds.

"You did great," I said. "How did it feel to move?"

"Not bad . . . not bad at all. I think I'm going to be okay."

"Well, of course you are. They brought lunch. Do you want to eat something?"

Blake's eyes softened. I rolled the tray table, positioned it over his knees, and tugged at the cellophane wrapper of a turkey sandwich. The patient ate slowly and deliberately, taking small morsels of food intermixed with sips of juice. A few minutes later—the food gone—my husband smiled.

* * *

Later, I returned to the motel to email family and friends regarding the morning's events.

Hi, All:

The cosmic forces have officially taken the reigns, so if you don't already, start believing in miracles. I left Blake for his midday nap in the ICU to the sounds of disbelief. All Blake's tubes are out (except for the peepee one, for convenience). He has gotten out of bed, taken a walk, and sat up to eat. The eating part involved a full meal, as in sandwich, soup, fruit, juice and a martini (just wanted to see if you were paying attention). His lungs are doing well and his oxygen count is way up. He can move the blue line on the spirometer to 1200+, where most patients can't go above 500 so soon after surgery. The physical therapist came in just before I left to talk about his first walk and subsequent exercises, only to find out we'd been there and done that.

"So, didn't you just have surgery yesterday?" she asked, looking at her pad, then at Blake. "You're Blake Webster, right?"

"Yeah, got out yesterday around noon," Blake said as he dutifully rotated his ankles and wiggled his toes.

Elaine aside: By the way . . . I like his shave. You should see his legs . . . smooth, round . . . well, better stop there.

"But, you look like most patients do after a week," she added with a glance at Blake's nurse.

"He's doing amazingly well. I haven't seen such progress in a long time . . . makes my job easy," she said with a shoulder shrug.

Bottom line: Not expecting such a quick recovery, they don't have a vacant room for us yet, but they may have one this afternoon, but more likely tomorrow. All this means is that he has to sleep in the ICU one more night and I only get a couple of hours more of visiting time today. On the other hand, I'll sleep better knowing that he's under constant surveillance for one more night.

Once we move, I'll be taking up most of the routine care—i.e., putting on my best nagging voice to keep him moving. The more he walks, exercises, and practices deep breathing the sooner we get to go home. There, the biggest challenge will be the simple exercise of getting in and out of bed. He can't use his arms to lift anything except food and water, and that includes pushing himself up.

His incision looks incredible. It's short with no redness or oozing. But he won't be able to drive or place any strain on it for three weeks. The usual length of full recovery is six months. For some reason, I'm thinking it will be more like two to three. Good work, doc.

Well, got to get back to the hospital. I'll send another update tomorrow.

Elaine

* * *

The afternoon crawled by. Blake napped—I read and wrote in my journal. While Blake had been in surgery, a dog-eared copy of Judith Guest's novel, *Ordinary People*, had summoned me from the waiting room bookshelf. I had seen the movie several times, but the book stuck in my hands like putty—I couldn't put it down.

The teaser on the back cover spoke to me.

> *These are the Jarretts: Calvin is a determined, successful, dutiful provider. Beth is an organized, efficient wife, still beautiful after 20 years of marriage. They had two sons, Conrad and Buck. Now they have one. They are ordinary people. And they are coming apart.*

The past few months had threatened to unravel our own lives. I took comfort in the story of a family struggling to find its way again. The author's insights into complex psychological issues, such as depression and post traumatic stress syndrome, caught my attention. I'd watched grieving families at bedsides, overheard stressful cellphone conversations in the hall, stumbled on sibling arguments about a loved one's care. I'd also seen heroic examples of love and support. It was all here, as if under a microscope.

At times I questioned the wisdom of my doing all this alone. Friends offered to come along. Why didn't I accept? Past hurts had left a deep-seated fear of emotional desertion by friends and family. I had lost faith and trust in people—something I wanted to regain—but I was too vulnerable right now and felt safer alone. I strived for control, where I had none. I could control myself, but other people were too unpredictable. So, I focused on Blake. He would be well and we would be all right; only then could I try and heal the past with the present.

We'd resigned ourselves to the fact that Blake would stay one more night in the ICU, so I learned how to work the TV remote and then showed Blake. After I left at six-thirty, when visiting hours were over, the remote control would be his friend for the night.

Then around five o'clock Blake's nurse delivered the good news. "You got lucky. We have a room available."

An orderly pushed over a wheelchair as I collected Blake's bag of stuff: clothes, a Sequoia Hospital water container with straw, a plastic vomit catcher, extra tissues—all the essentials. The orderly lowered Blake into the chair, I set the parcel on his lap, and off we went to the Cardiac Surveillance Unit (CSU). We had graduated.

Room with a View

"I'm sorry about the room location. Being across from the elevators can be noisy," the ICU nurse remarked as she rolled her passenger into a small private room.

"Well, it's not the Hilton, but at least you have the place to yourself," I said. "Nice view of the construction site, too," I added, trying to be funny.

Sequoia Hospital, built in 1950, was receiving an upgrade. A new medical center was under construction right below us. A giant yellow crane hovered over the steel skeleton of a four-story structure. Hard-hatted workers scurried below like ants.

"There used to be trees out there—now it's a sea of concrete. Well, that's progress," the nurse said as she helped Blake into bed. "I'll be right back. And I'll get your CSU nurse."

I looked around our new home and decided it would do fine—as if we had a choice. Natural light streamed in through the picture window, and a TV hovered above us on the institutional-pink wall. A white board with six cartoon faces, ranging from happy to sad, hung on the wall across from Blake's bed. There was a sink area, a tray table, extra chair, private bathroom. I took a deep breath, exhaled, and piled my laptop and purse on the floor in the corner.

The two women returned. "This is Nurse Sun, your CSU nurse. She'll explain the routine. I've got to get back to the ICU. Good luck." And with a wave she was gone.

Of all Blake's nurses, Nurse Sun was our favorite. A petite, high-energy Asian woman, she had a demeanor that matched her name. She understood about proper diet, exercise, and even yoga. Though her accent was occasionally difficult to penetrate, overall communication was good. Both Blake and I were glad she was in charge of our orientation. She educated us about hospital procedures and took us on our first walk.

"Seven o'clock. Will you be all right if I leave now?" I asked, hoping for an affirmative answer. I was beyond tired, wanted to get out of that hospital, yet felt guilty asking.

"Oh, sure . . . you go ahead. I think I might be able to doze off for awhile now."

I gathered up my belongings, set them on the chair, and gently hugged my husband and his chest pillow. "During the night, just pretend that pillow is me," I quipped. "I'll be here in spirit."

Survival Tips for a Successful Hospital Stay:

- Use the white board to track pain levels. In a prominent section of wall space hangs a large white board, several colored markers, and an eraser. Normally it includes the Wong-Baker FACES Pain Rating Scale. This is a series of six cartoon faces. The first is smiling; the last is crying. The others range from worried to frowning. The scale ranges from zero=no hurt, two=hurts a bit, four=hurts little more, six=hurts even more, eight=hurts a lot, and ten=hurts worst. Frequently ask about the extent of your patient's discomfort. Write the time and date beneath the appropriate picture. One glance at the board tells a busy nurse if your patient's medications require adjustment.
- Stay ahead of the pain. I asked Blake at least once an hour how he felt and watched his body language. Knowing my husband, I had an innate sense of his pain tolerance. If he indicated distress, or looked more uncomfortable than usual, I'd ask that he have another

dose of Oxycodone or Tylenol.

▪ Routinely at shift changes, a new nurse will write his or her name on the white board. If not, ask the nurse to do so, or do it yourself. This fosters familiarity, and allows you to track care levels and verbally delivered information. Jot down questions and any reminders about follow-up care. Document conflicting information or instructions so that they are readily available when the doctor visits on rounds.

▪ Your patient will have a central-line catheter, a small tube placed in a large vein to draw blood and give fluids. If you notice any changes in skin color or redness around the insertion, immediately alert the nurse.

▪ Wash your hands often with soap and warm water. Rub your hands together for fifteen seconds, rinse well, and dry. Use the containers of hand sanitizers available throughout the hospital. Rub the sanitizer over your hands and allow it to dry. Ask your patient and any visitors to do the same.

▪ Limit visitors, especially sick ones. The last thing you need is for you or your patient to catch a chest cold or flu. It's wonderful for you and your patient to feel the love of family and friends, but a hospital stay is stressful and tiring. In today's electronic world, it's easier than ever to stay in touch remotely. Sequoia Hospital has CarePages, which are secured personal websites set up and managed by the patient or caregiver. Invited guests are able to keep in touch with messages and photos. I set my laptop up on Blake's tray table. As messages came in, I would read them to him. In turn we would compose replies together—we stayed connected without the added stress of entertaining visitors. Consider meeting well wishers for coffee or lunch. That way, you and the patient both get a deserved break.

▪ Emphasize walking, an important part of recovery. Two post-surgery risks, blood clots in the legs and pneumonia, can be avoided by getting your patient out of bed at regular intervals. The first walk will be with a nurse. If all goes well, you can then accompany the patient on walks. Never let the patient walk alone. Blake had a portable vital-sign monitor attached with electrodes to his chest that transmitted to the computer at the nurses' station. Any unusual cardiac activity would be noticed immediately, but a slip or fall may not.

▪ Alternate rest periods with activity. A physical therapist will provide written instructions for General Lower Extremity Exercises. His or her daily visits will include assisted exercise periods. Afterward, it's your job as caregiver to see that the patient practices ankle pumps, quad and hamstring exercises, sitting knee bending, and leg raises. Alternate bed rest, sitting, and walking. Your patient should not sit for more than forty-five minutes without a walk. Get your patient out of bed for all meals, and every day increase the number of walks. Distance and speed are not an issue—movement is what's important.

▪ Continue the breathing exercises. Keep the spirometer (a plastic instrument that is blown into to measure lung capacity) handy and use it often. The patient should breathe from the belly several times, relax, then with more shallow breaths blow into the spirometer. Write the readings on your white board with the date and time.

- Encourage coughing after surgery, which will help remove mucous from the lungs. A small pillow held tightly against the chest incision will alleviate discomfort. At least four times a day, the patient should take ten deep breaths then cough twice. This is a good practice to continue for at least two weeks.
- Watch Hospital Education TV. Sequoia Hospital's version is "On Demand ED TV," with programming geared toward the recuperating patient. Blake and I watched several shows together and it gave us a feeling that we weren't alone, that many others shared our concerns and challenges. Some of the more informative titles included: "What You Need to Know About Your Cardiac Surgery," "Heart Failure—Eating to Feel Better," and "Taking Care of Yourself after Heart Surgery."

Chapter Eight
Sleepless in Redwood City

Saturday Night without a Date

My footsteps echoed in the dimly lit parking garage until I reached my car. I wasn't used to this. I could do it—be alone—but I didn't like it. I liked getting in the passenger seat, letting Blake take the wheel. I can rely on him to find the fastest route from point A to point B with the fewest red lights. On my own, I always choose a slower, safer direction, and tonight was no exception. Rather than risk a left turn on the main thoroughfare, I drove the side streets back to the motel. I'd set the radio preset for San Francisco's classic rock station, KFOG. Blind Faith's "Can't Find My Way Home" broke the silence. I turned it up and sang along.

I pulled into the motel parking lot and found most spots taken. Popular place, I thought. I parked around back and lugged my laptop up to the room. Once inside I realized that the thin walls allowed me to hear most of what was going on with the neighbors. Music and telephone conversations reverberated though the wall; through the other I could hear repeated thumpings, followed by a telltale squeal and subsequent laughter. In no mood to listen to sexual pleasure, I clicked the TV remote and turned up the volume. I surfed the channels, found nothing worth watching, and dialed in QVC, the home shopping channel. If nothing else, it offered me happy, animated people. Hell, maybe I'd find a pair of shoes I liked.

I set up my laptop, hit the power switch, and headed for the makeshift kitchen. I found the container of chicken noodle soup I'd bought at the Whole Foods Deli and set it in the microwave. As the soup heated, I sliced some cheese and sourdough bread, dished salad, and poured a glass of Port. I congratulated myself on having the foresight to bring three bottles of St. Francis Winery's Port, a kind of vertical tasting—vintage years of 2007, 2008 and 2009. Blake had shared some with me the night before his surgery, and he thought it helped him sleep; I would finish them off over the next three nights.

I ate dinner cross-legged on the bed and marveled at the turquoise jewelry that the TV show host pitched with such gusto. A middle-aged woman, she of the heavy make-up, long manicured nails, and silver bracelets, called the ring she wore "the deal of a lifetime." It must have been true because they were selling out. I almost rushed to my laptop to buy one online, but stopped myself, knowing it would only be a "comfort" buy. It was especially foolish in my case because except for my wedding band, I wore no rings.

I laughed out loud. *Women and their shopping habits. Whether scared, nervous, happy, or sad, just go shopping and all will be right in the world. Ha!*

After dinner, I ran a hot bath. As I soaked, tensions drifting away in the warm water and port wine, I relaxed enough to consider sleep. By ten o'clock I turned off the TV and got under the covers. But menopausal hot flashes kept me alternating between hot and cold, and I got up several times to adjust the heater. Without Blake next to me, I sprawled out, but couldn't get comfortable. Every half hour I glanced at the clock until I finally drifted off around two a.m.

Sunday Morning—Care for the Caregiver

The next morning I awoke with most of the covers on the floor and my head at the foot of the bed—I had no idea how I got that way. It was still early, six a.m., and I started a pot of coffee. As I brushed my teeth I wondered how to kill the two and a half hours before I could go back to the hospital. I remembered the exercise DVD I'd packed and smiled. I could get a workout and get even with my neighbors by cranking up the sound at this early hour. *I'll show you thumping*, I thought. *I hope you have hangovers*.

For the next 30 minutes, I sweated and grunted to Jackie Warner's *Xtreme Timesaver Training*. Afterwards, rejuvenated, I jumped in the shower. I hadn't heard a peep from my neighbors.

After cleaning up, I slipped on my bathrobe and settled on the bed for morning meditation. I pushed a pillow under me, crossed my legs and straightened my back against the coolness of the wall. The instant I closed my eyes, I felt calmness wash over me. I recited a protective blessing conjured from my Catholic background.

"In the name of the Father, The Son, and the Holy Spirit, Amen."

I wondered why I continued to say those words. Maybe it was like comfort food you remember from childhood. No matter where you are, just the thought of it brings joy.

I meditated for an hour, letting thoughts drift in and out of my mind without disturbance. I'd notice them and let them go. Mostly I watched the light show behind my eyelids as I focused on the point above and between my eyes. I used the breathing patterns taught by the Self Realization Fellowship lessons to take me deeper into stillness. The combination of exercise, physical cleansing, and meditation gave me a renewed determination.

* * *

A Brief Encounter with Dr. Kardon

Blake smelled the coffee I was carrying before he saw me. "I thought you might like some real coffee, instead of that brown water they give you," I said. I pulled his tray table over to the side of the bed and set two insulated paper cups down.

"You look good this morning . . . how do you feel?" I asked.

"Not too bad, but I can't sleep here. Even when I get comfortable and start to drift off, someone comes in and wakes me up. The nurses check every room every hour, and they always want to do something to me." Blake reached for one of the cups, then looked at me and smiled weakly. "Thanks for the coffee. It smells great."

"Have you had breakfast? Want me to get you something from the cafeteria?"

"No thanks. They brought cereal and whole-wheat toast."

As I took a sip of my coffee, two men in white hospital shirts approached the open door. I realized it was Dr. Kardon accompanied by a physician's assistant, whose name tag read: Taemin Surh.

Dr. Kardon spoke only to the assistant, not to us. He rattled off the details of Blake's surgery and said he had atrial fibrillation and would need Coumadin. Blake, haltingly, tried to cut in.

"Dr. Gaudiani—"

"I'm not Dr. Gaudiani. I'm Dr. Kardon. If I was Dr. Gaudiani, I'd be a whole lot richer and somewhere else on a Sunday." I looked for a smile, a touch of irony, but found neither.

"Sorry," Blake said, "but I don't understand what you're saying about the fibrillation and Coumadin."

"I'm not convinced he needs Coumadin. His heart seems to be settling down," Taemin Surh put in.

"Look. I don't want to argue about this. He's in A-fib and I'm prescribing Coumadin, subject closed. Let's go."

And before Blake or I could say anything else, the two men left, with nary a wave or nod.

"That was cold," I said. "Look, we'll find out about this Coumadin thing. Don't worry. Let's not think about it now."

Physical Therapy

Nurse Sun got wind that Blake's physical therapist, Terry, was on rounds and followed her into Blake's room. The nurse seemed to have a sixth sense when someone was fiddling with her patients, and she came in to keep an eye on the therapy session.

As Terry exchanged pleasantries with Blake, I squeezed myself into a corner, out of the way. Nurse Sun stood at the foot of Blake's bed—silent and stolid.

Terry ignored the observers and focused on her patient. "Okay, Blake, let's get you out of bed. How are you doing with that?"

"It hurts to move," Blake said.

"Well, move we must. Now swing your legs over and I'll support your weight . . . then stand."

After a few tries, Blake got to his feet. I looked at Nurse Sun. Her face showed concern, but she remained silent. Blake, too, looked concerned. As Terry took Blake through his exercises, I worried it was too much, too soon, but the physical therapist, though gentle, persisted. Twenty minutes later, Blake fell back into bed, exhausted. Terry reminded Blake to do that routine three times a day, handed me a page of instructions, and scurried off.

Blake looked at Nurse Sun. "I'm tired. Do I have to do all of that two more times today?"

The nurse took the papers from me and shook her head no. "It's too much for today. I want you to walk more and do the exercises you can do in bed. Replace the squats and toe raises with extra walks to prevent blood clots, but don't push so hard."

Nurse Sun's beeper vibrated and she clicked it off. Well, if you're okay for now, I've got to go next door . . . call me if you need me . . . I'm right down the hall."

General Lower Extremity Exercises for the First Few Days after Surgery:

- Ankle Pumps. While lying or sitting, move your foot backward and forward, and rotate your ankle in circles at least ten times.
- Quad sets. While lying flat on back, squeeze and tighten the thigh muscle as you push your knee into the mattress.
- Heel Slides. On your back, bend each knee and bring your heel up close to your buttocks, then lower. Alternate legs and do as many reps as feel comfortable.
- Sitting exercises. Sitting upright in a chair, 1) lift your foot until your lower leg is parallel with the floor; hold for a few seconds, then lower it back down. Do five reps with each leg. 2) Keeping your leg bent, raise one leg at a time off the chair, as high as possible, hold for a few seconds, lower, and repeat with each leg.
- Walking. Try not to sit for more than forty-five minutes at a time. Increase the length and frequency of your walks a little each day.

▪ Listen to your body. Each person's recovery time is different. Push yourself, but not to exhaustion. Document each walk and all completed exercises on your white board. Remember that an early discharge date depends on steady progress. You will be released when your pain is manageable, you can walk without assistance five to six times a day, you can get in and out of bed without using your arms, and you've had a bowel movement. Tell your doctor about any bloated feelings or swelling of the feet or ankles. Edema may indicate that your heart isn't effectively pumping blood.

Sunday Strolls and Goodnight Kisses

Hi All,

Live from Redwood City, it's Sunday afternoon.

Well, we've settled into the executive suite. The fog burned off around noon and the sun is streaming in. Construction is underway for a new hospital wing, and a giant yellow steel crane stands guard outside our window. Behind mounds of gravel are redwoods—deep green against the pale blue sky. Redwood City is a pretty place. Each morning I drive through pristine neighborhoods, I make a left at the white picket fence, right onto Jefferson St., past the Tudor style apartment buildings, right on Hudson through several four-way stops, slowing for the occasional jogger or dog walker, and then left on Whipple. The hospital sits atop "Cardiac Hill," a climb that rivals San Francisco's finest. Some mornings I trek it, for a workout. Otherwise, I chat with the shuttle bus driver as I'm chauffeured to the top.

At 9:00 this morning, Blake was awake and alert when I arrived. A few minutes later, Dr. Kardon stopped by on rounds with a physician's assistant. I don't care for Dr. Kardon much. Steve will relate, when I say that he reminds me of Bud. (An egotistical character in one of my memoir chapters.) I'm sure he's competent, but he seems too full of himself. Doesn't stay long. He talks around us, instead of to us—show off.

Soon Nurse Sun comes in. Yes, that's really her name Myung Sun, a petite, fit, thirty-something Asian with an engaging smile, struggling English, and tons of patience. We like her. She checks vital signs and accompanies us on our first walk of the day. All is good so far, until Terry, the physical therapist appears. She's sweet, but somewhat overzealous in her approach. The heel-raises and semi-squats take their toll on Blake, and when she leaves we order more pain meds. Sun and I agree—too much, too soon. I'll keep an eye.

The problem with extra pain meds is that they make Blake nauseous, a feeling he abhors. Sun has a medication remedy delivered intravenously that takes away the nausea, but makes the patient sleepy. Napping during the day is frowned upon—better to return to normal sleep patterns soon. Blake pushes lunch away. (I couldn't recognize most of it and requested a sandwich for tomorrow in lieu of secret sauce chicken.)

Once we were feeling better, we checked email and I deleted the spam and unnecessary exchanges from Blake's inbox. We logged in to our revenue producers and were pleased to find activity. All the better for paying those insurance co-pays.

We got Blake out of bed without assistance at 1:00 and took our third walk of the day. We practiced several techniques for re-entry and finally found one that worked. (The key is plopping the butt down as far north as possible before dropping to the side, bending the knees and lifting the legs.) Success.

Right now I'm letting him nap—to hell with perfect sleep patterns. Oops, an orderly's here with a wheelchair. Time for a chest x-ray? Seems weird, but Blake, now awake, hops aboard. Nurse Sun, sensing something askew, appears at our door. When I explain where her patient went, she jumps on the phone. "Get Blake Webster back to his bed. No x-ray until Tuesday." Minutes later Blake rolled back in, pushed by an apologetic orderly. Nurse Sun, satisfied that all was as it should be, smiles, waves, and continues her rounds.

I'll touch base again tomorrow.

Love, Elaine

I stayed with Blake until late Sunday evening. We had taken a total of six walks and two meals together. The hospital food, except for the mystery chicken, was not bad. I brought myself salads from the cafeteria and finished off what Blake didn't like on his plate. We watched TV, mainly CNN news, and I let him nap on and off as I wrote emails and poetry. Around nine p.m. I snuggled up to my sore, sponge-bathed husband with his three-day growth of beard. Four clear plastic tubes dangled from his neck. Remnants of sticky tape marked where chest tubes had been. My heart ached for him. He looked like he'd recently emerged from a war zone.

I gave Blake's shoulders a squeeze. "I'm beat. I think I'll go."

Blake's sad eyes foreshadowed what he was about to say. "I want to go home. Take me home."

"Soon, honey . . . soon. Now try and get some sleep. I'll be back early tomorrow. I want to be here when the doctor makes his rounds."

I squeezed in the elevator with three new dads coming down from the third-floor maternity ward. I regularly shared the ride with proud fathers lugging teddy bears and flower bouquets. Tonight, after a long day of caring for their spouses, they looked as tired as I felt. As a writer, I conjured up stories about them. In their future, I saw shiny new bicycles for Christmas, high-school graduations, weddings, anniversaries . . . I thought about infants becoming toddlers, learning to walk, and then run. I said a silent prayer for each—that life would give them and their families the best of everything. I wished their lives to be care-free and painless—knowing too well the impossibility of that.

The ding of the elevator bell jarred me from my thoughts, and I stepped out into the florescent-lighted hallway. Directly across from the elevator was a wall of pictures of hospital donors. I stopped to look at the names and faces. In a journalistic mood, I took out my flip pad and made some notes. A passerby kept throwing glances my way, and I could only imagine what she was thinking: terrorist? stalker? contract killer? Half expecting her to call security, I dropped pencil and pad in my purse and walked on, my imagination percolating.

Great names on those walls . . . perfect for my next short-story collection. Take Gladys Hopsinger, a granny, photographed in designer glasses and pearls. Last year she donated hundreds of thousands of dollars to the new hospital wing. Where did she get it? I bet she married a rich old man when she was in her twenties, killed him off, and took up with the gardener, who is now her book agent. Hmmm.

Chapter Nine
Monday Morning and It Sure Looks Fine

Taemin—Bearer of Good News

Taemin Surh arrived on Monday morning rounds without Dr. Kardon. Sunshine illuminated the room as we exchanged pleasantries with the physician assistant. I noticed that his body language had changed—soft eyes, gentle smile, calm and clear.

He flipped through Blake's medical chart. "So I see here that they administered Coumadin last night—"

Blake pounced on that one. "The nurse brought it last night after Elaine left. I told her I wasn't sure about it. She called Dr. Castro (another cardiac surgeon at PCCVS), and he said he was familiar with my case and that I should have it . . . so I took it."

"Hmm. Okay, fine," Taemin responded. "So, how do you feel?"

"Like I want to go home. Can I?" Blake chuckled, not expecting a positive response.

Taemin looked at the white board, where I'd recorded our walks—two already that morning. He placed a stethoscope to Blake's chest and back. "Well the heart murmur's gone. It appears they fixed you. You might be able to go home tomorrow."

"You're kidding, right? So soon? That would be great. When will we know?" Blake spewed out the words in one breath.

Taemin crossed his arms and leaned against the window ledge. "Whoa. Slow down . . . I said maybe. If you keep improving . . . well, let's wait until morning to decide. And keep taking the Coumadin."

Blake locked his gaze onto mine, and I saw the errant sparkle return.

"Well, if there's nothing else, I'll be going." Taemin slipped around the bed, squeezed past me, and headed out the door.

"Wow! Great news," I said. "That'd be so cool if we could leave tomorrow. Are you sure you're ready?"

"I am more than ready. I want to take a real shower and get some sleep. If something comes up we can always call Dr. Erickson. It's not like we'll be without medical advice."

I cut Blake off mid-sentence. "Oh, I forgot to tell you. I talked to your brother last night, and he's going to come by today to see you and take me to lunch. That's okay . . . right?"

"I guess so. No, I mean, that's fine. It'll be good to see him and you could use the break."

Something in Blake's tone suggested it wasn't all right, but I brushed it aside. I did need a break and Brad's always been a good friend to me. I was looking forward to seeing him.

A Friendly Face—Lunch with Brad

I looked up from my laptop computer screen to see the mini-version of Blake slip into the room. The two brothers share similar features, but Brad's ten years younger and much shorter—a result of pre-teen surgery for scoliosis that left him with a fused spine. We joke about how it's the stubborn gene that overcomes the rest of the bad heredity—Webster toughness.

Brad greeted us in his usual manner. "Hi, guys. How's it going?"

With Brad, what you see is what you get—no hidden agendas. I like that. Blake and Brad share the gift of gab. Normally I wouldn't be able to get a word in edgewise, but Blake was less chatty than usual. Brad generally picked up the slack. I kept a close eye on my husband as his brother cheerily chatted about this and that: his job, his wife Mary Ann, her job, my job, the weather—typical hospital visitor stuff.

I let fifteen to twenty minutes pass before I tapped my watch. "We should get going . . . I'm starved, and I don't want to leave our boy alone too long."

I kissed Blake on the forehead and grabbed my jacket and my brother-in-law. Out in the hall I thumped the elevator button and turned to Brad. "So, he looks good, doesn't he?"

"Yeah, he does—better than I thought."

* * *

I chose a restaurant I'd discovered that morning while searching for the local post office. Blake's illness had crimped his business's cash flow and I'd been waiting to mail some bill payments. That morning the county had direct deposited my paycheck and so I sent the payments on their way. As I circled back toward the hospital, a casual patisserie caught my eye, so I suggested it to Brad. Besides French-style bakery fare, they served casual lunch items, wine and beer. I ordered a smoked-salmon sandwich and Brad followed my lead.

"Something to drink?" the clerk asked.

"I'd sure love a beer," I answered, feeling mischievous. "Brad?"

"Twist my arm." Brad laughed, held out his arm, and I twisted it affectionately.

We took our food and drinks to a window table, and for the first time in days I let out a sigh of relief.

"I feel like I've been holding my breath," I said.

"You've been through a lot. I'm glad I came down. You shouldn't be doing this all alone. I wanted to be sure you were okay."

I took a sip of beer and continued breathing from my belly. "I don't know where to turn these days. I feel dis-connected. Maybe it started with all I went through at work. I dunno, but I'm having a hard time trusting."

"Has it gotten any better there? Is that boss still harassing you?"

"Oh, she's backed off some . . . had to . . . it was too obvious. Someone must have said something to her about it. But something else has happened . . . I can't put my finger on it. It's like my world has gone askew somehow. This heart stuff has understandably changed Blake . . . he's become distant. I've been trying to cope by writing. As long as I'm at the keyboard, I'm happy . . . well, content. But then last Friday, the people in my memoir group—people I thought were my friends—they changed too. I dunno, maybe it's all me. Maybe I'm nuts."

"You're not nuts—you're going through more than you can handle, that's all. And like I said, you shouldn't try and do it all alone. People do care about you. Mary Ann and I care. She insisted I come see you."

I took a bite of my sandwich and another sip of beer. I could feel myself relax. I was so glad Brad had come. I felt safe with him—I opened up more than usual.

"You know, I want to trust people . . . I really do. But each time I go all out, take chances, show any vulnerability, they sneak up on me and pounce. My alternative is to appear tough, but it's not my way. I'm so tired of people telling me to toughen up, face my fears, and stand up to the bullies. My answer is that the bullies should stop bullying. Does that make any sense?"

"I know how you feel. But you can't hide—they're everywhere."

Brad's simple statement said it all. That's what I love about him—simple wisdom. We ate for awhile in comfortable silence and I reflected on the past few years. What had changed? When did I go from happy-go-lucky to an I'm-not-sure-I-can-cope-with-this type of person? I watched through the window as a city bus let out its passengers. I noticed that no one spoke or smiled as they disembarked. Several pulled out cell phones or began text messaging on handheld electronic devices.

I wondered: *Does anyone feel comfortable?*

Halfway though our beers, the conversation lightened. I began to relax and liked hearing about Brad's and Mary Ann's recent vacation in Hawaii. We compared island stories and gossiped about family and friends. By the time we rose to leave, I felt better.

After lunch, Brad and I returned to the hospital. The moment we entered Blake's room, I could feel his tension.

"That was a long lunch," he said, an edge to his tone. "I've been waiting for you, so I could take another walk." Blake's sparkle was gone; in its place: worry lines.

Brad took the cue, gathered his things, gave me a hug, and wished his brother a quick recovery. I waited until I heard him get in the elevator before addressing my husband.

"We weren't gone that long. Is everything okay?"

"I'm trying to stay on schedule . . . that's all, and I can't walk without someone with me."

As I helped Blake out of bed, I thought about what the Mended Hearts volunteer had said about the infamous third day after surgery. She told us that it takes a couple of days before the body processes the recent trauma; often the patient becomes angry. She said it's like the body is "pissed off" about what just happened to it. Blake, however, was more impatient than angry. As we took our walk around the floor, I coaxed him to talk about how he felt.

"You're looking more tired this afternoon. Are you sure we should be thinking about going home?"

"I am tired—and bored and sore. All I can think about is going home. Tonight, like last night, I won't be able to sleep. When you're not here, I stare at the TV or the wall. Time ticks by—every minute feels like an hour."

"Would it help if I brought you something to read, or I could bring your laptop and you could write or surf the Internet or—"

Blake snapped me off. "No, I can't concentrate. I don't know if it's the medications or what, but I can't think clearly. I'm so frustrated."

My attempt to cheer was going nowhere, so I quit trying. That afternoon, I think we both stopped trying. All we could do was wait—not easy for us, the "surge ahead team." But wait we did. Then about six o'clock I called it quits.

"Sweetie . . . I need to go. I can't sit still anymore. Do you want to take one more walk before I go?"

"No, I'm done for the day. Could you fill my water and hand me the remote control"

I did as instructed, then propped Blake up as best I could. I gave him a kiss and a hug and left. Once outside, I took a deep breath of cold air and zipped my jacket. A prayer went out to the universe: *Please let us go home, please let us go home . . .*

Asleep at Last

For the rest of the evening, I felt like a character in a *Twilight Zone* episode, where the same day repeats over and over—for eternity. My motel-room routine was well established by now: shower, eat, read, and send emails. At ten o'clock I set a glass of port on the bed stand, turned on and muted QVC, and crawled into bed.

I reopened *Ordinary People*. Rereading a snatch of dialog between the Conrad character and his date, Jeannine, I was struck by the ability of the author to capture complex feelings in simple sentences. I thought about Steve Boga, my editor and friend, who taught me that. With writing, less is more. I threw off the covers and went to the computer and typed the section into an email and sent it to him. I half expected he'd be there at the other end, but how could he be at that hour?

Feeling momentarily desolate, I began to cry. It was like a release of all the pain, hurt, and disappointment I'd ever had in my life. I let every demon flow out in huge sobs. Then, finally exhausted, I slipped into bed, turned out the light, threw the book across the room, and fell into a comatose sleep.

Overcoming Depression and De-Stressing

- *Postoperative patient depression.* Emotional ups and downs are a normal part of recovery from heart surgery. If clinical depression has been an issue prior to surgery, be sure the patient continues close contact with his or her therapist. For patients who have never suffered from depression, these feelings may come as a surprise.
- *Caregiver depression.* You will have feelings of helplessness—this is normal. Taking care of a patient is often like caring for a child, sometimes even more difficult. You will not have answers to emotional questions like: When will this end? When will I feel whole again? When can I start doing the things I've always done? You can and should reassure the patient, but your words may fall on deaf ears. I tried to stay in the moment, while reminding myself that this too will pass. That life will be good again, even better than ever, and that helped.
- *Problem solving.* Break day-to-day problems down to their simplest terms, and use creative thinking to find solutions. Solicit help to complete errands. Schedule your time for patient care and for down time. If you feel overwhelmed, find a way to rest. Your health is as important as the patient's.

▪ *Communicate your feelings to others.* Suppressed frustration has been linked to adverse health conditions. Be clear about your feelings without blaming yourself or others for them. Look to spiritual practices or religious beliefs to help you put life into perspective and appropriately control your feelings. Assert yourself by insisting that your emotional needs are met.

▪ *Let it out.* It's okay to cry. The all-out cry I sometimes allowed myself released weeks of suppressed tension and pent-up emotion. Choose a safe place to be alone, then cry; throw things, yell, jump up and down—whatever works for you. Don't break Aunt Jane's Ming Dynasty vase or physically hurt yourself, but allow the feelings out—get rid of them. If it helps, write them down, then crumple them up and throw them away; tear the paper into pieces or throw it in a fireplace. You can and will move on.

▪ *Minimize stress in your life.* Are you easily angered? You may be blowing things out of proportion. Get all the facts before jumping to negative conclusions. Are you insecure about your abilities? Take classes, or find a mentor that can help you succeed in your work and your personal life. Overwhelmed with responsibilities? Decide what has to be done and learn to say no to the rest. Feeling tense? Exercise, meditate, read, write, get a massage, or take a long hot bath with no interruptions. Upset with others? Use "I" statements to express your needs and concerns. Forget about trying to change others—change yourself.

▪ *Be kind to yourself and your patient.* Greet both the good days and the bad days with a smile. Major surgery is never easy, but time does indeed heal. Help yourself and the patient to spread activities throughout the week. Don't do hours of errands one day only to find you both exhausted the next. The key is to move forward in increments and not push too hard. It will get easier.

Chapter Ten
Tuesday Getaway

It's Complicated—Coumadin—the Movie

The sun was shining, and I was energized by the idea of going home. The second I saw Blake, I blurted, "I got here early. Didn't want to miss the doctor. Heard anything yet?"

"Nothing yet," Blake said. "Could you pull the tray table over? I'm going to get up to eat. Breakfast should be here soon."

I set Blake up as he asked, and soon an orderly came in and set down a food tray. As Blake ate scrambled eggs and toast, a pharmacist appeared to talk about his Coumadin regimen. He handed me two brochures detailing the drug therapy and the role of Vitamin K and Coumadin.

"So, has anyone explained all this to you yet?" the pharmacist asked.

"Barely. I'm already taking it, and I know it's because of the A-fib, but I don't know much more," Blake said.

"We keep asking about the drug, but no one seems to want to elaborate," I added.

"Well, Coumadin—generic name warfarin sodium—is a blood thinner. When your heart's atrium quivers as a result of surgery, it is a potential site for blood clots. If a blood clot breaks free and travels to the brain, it can cause a stroke, so we administer Coumadin to keep the blood thin and less likely to clot."

"We keep hearing about lifestyle changes—what does that mean?" I asked.

"Read through this literature, then watch the educational program on TV. It will answer most of your questions. If you don't understand something, ask your doctor when he comes around later. I urge you to follow the routine. One of the pharmacists here thought he could bypass Coumadin, and he had a stroke. He knew the risks and ignored them. It doesn't make sense."

After the pharmacist left, we read the brochures and watched the TV program. Before long we felt like experts on the do's and don'ts of the therapy.

Coumadin Therapy

- Coumadin is a life saver, with risks. As a blood thinner, Coumadin can cause bleeding problems. Be alert for: pain or swelling of the abdomen or limbs, headaches, dizziness or weakness, unexplained bruising, nosebleeds, bleeding gums, pink or brown urine, red or black stools, unusually heavy menstrual flow, coughing up blood, and vomiting blood or material that resembles coffee grounds.
- Vitamins, herbal supplements, and some medications interact negatively with Coumadin. Be certain your physician has a current list of medicines you take.
- Do not take Coumadin if you have bleeding problems, are pregnant, or are allergic to warfarin.
- Do not drink alcohol while taking Coumadin.

▪ The major inconvenience for Coumadin patients is that they are required to have regular blood tests (PT/INR tests). A drop of blood from a finger prick is all that's required to test your PT/INR levels. Afterward, you must follow the regimen exactly as prescribed. You will begin with weekly monitoring. If your level stabilizes, you may be able to test less often.

▪ Vitamin K can interfere with the blood-thinning effects of Coumadin. You can eat foods high in Vitamin K, but you must maintain a consistent average of these foods in your diet. Leafy green vegetables, such as kale, parsley, spinach, broccoli, and brussel sprouts, are rich in Vitamin K. Stay away from cranberry products. Your doctor will provide you with a list of Vitamin K levels in common foods.

▪ Cuts and injuries can be more dangerous than usual. Avoid sports that put you at risk for bumps and bruises. If you fall, hit your head, or cut yourself, seek immediate medical attention. Skin necrosis or gangrene is the most serious of the side effects. If you notice skin discoloration to any area of your body, see your doctor right away. Purple Toe Syndrome is another serious condition. Do not ignore the signs.

As we finished watching the educational program, a woman came into our room and announced she was our nutritionist. She left more brochures for us to read and suggested we watch one more educational program on nutrition while we awaited discharge.

Heart Health and Nutrition

- Reduce sodium intake. Strive to eat less than 1500 milligrams of sodium per day. Remember that one teaspoon of salt contains 2300 milligrams of sodium, so put that salt shaker away. The American Heart Association is encouraging food manufacturers and restaurants to reduce sodium levels by half over the next ten years. You need to start today. Read labels and eat fresh.
- Strive for low fat and low cholesterol. Only animal products contain cholesterol. Have your blood tested regularly for HDL (good cholesterol) and LDL (bad cholesterol). Ideally, your total cholesterol should be less than 200 mg/dl, with the LDL level less than 70 mg/dl and the HDL level at 40 mg/dl or greater. Stay away from high-fat foods. Saturated fats and trans fats raise your cholesterol and contribute to clogged arteries and heart disease. Monounsaturated and polyunsaturated fats are healthier alternatives and can lower cholesterol. Remember that all fats are calorie rich, and oils are all fat.
- Control your weight. When calories consumed equal calories expended, your weight stabilizes. If you need to lose weight, decrease intake and increase activity. Forget fad diets, and focus on portion sizes and food quality. Small changes will bring weight-loss success over time. Starvation diets slow metabolism as your body holds on to fat stores for sustenance. Stay away from caffeinated diet supplements. They will raise your blood pressure and put you at greater risk for heart attack and stroke.

- Eat fresh and enjoy at least five servings of fruits and vegetables every day. Eat whole grains and little or no red meat. Substitute lower-fat proteins, such as soy products, poultry, and fish.
- If you smoke, stop. Smoking increases the risk of coronary heart disease. Smoking robs you of some of your good cholesterol, boosts blood pressure, and increases the chance of blood clots and stroke. According to the Centers for Disease Control, cigarettes contain at least 250 chemicals harmful to your health and contribute to more than one in five deaths in the U.S.

We're Outta Here—Elaine Takes the Wheel

I looked at my watch for what seemed like the millionth time. Hoping to go home, I'd already checked out of the motel room. It was almost noon.

"When do daily rounds start? Isn't someone usually here by now?" I asked Blake.

"Usually. I'm going to call the nurse."

Blake hit the call button on the remote control, and in a few minutes a stocky young woman appeared. "Do you need something?" she asked.

"Do you know when the doctor will be here? I'm supposed to go home today, but I need to be discharged."

"I don't have any orders saying you're going home. Are

you sure it's today? We need to remove the central line . . . but I can't do that without doctor's orders."

"Can you call Dr. Gaudiani's office and find out? The physician's assistant, Taemin Surh, said he'd be by this morning and if nothing changed that he'd discharge me."

The urgency in Blake's voice persuaded the nurse to make the phone call, but she came back with little news. physician assistant Wilson Kee was behind on his rounds, but he would get to Blake as soon as he could. An hour later, I was pacing the floor when Wilson came into the room.

"Sorry I'm so late, but I'm covering double patients today. Plus you've been doing so well, I pushed our visit back some."

Wilson opened Blake's chart, but before he could read a word, Blake jumped in. "Taemin said yesterday I could be discharged today, and we were hoping to leave before the commute traffic got too bad."

Wilson ran his finger down Blake's chart. I held my breath.

"Discharge? No one told me about a discharge. Are you sure?"

"Yes . . . yes, I'm sure. He said if nothing changed, I could go home. I want to go home today," Blake pleaded.

Wilson pulled a chair up to the tray table, sat down, and flipped through the paperwork. "Well, I guess you can go. You need the central line out . . . and I'll have to write prescriptions. And you're on Coumadin. You have to have your levels tested again tomorrow. Where do you live?"

"Santa Rosa," I cut in. "Dr. Joel Erickson is his cardiologist. We can call his office for an appointment. We really don't want to stay another day."

As Wilson pulled out his prescription pad and discharge sheets, I found Dr. Erickson's phone number and Blake called his office.

"Tia? This is Blake Webster . . . yes, I'm doing good. If they let me go today, can I come in for a Coumadin test tomorrow? . . . a clinic? . . . that's perfect . . . thanks . . . bye."

Blake turned to Wilson. "Well, it's all set. Dr. Erickson has a Wednesday Coumadin clinic and we can go first thing tomorrow morning. Is that good enough?"

Wilson said nothing, just kept flipping through Blake's chart. Then he pulled his stethoscope from his pocket and listened to Blake's heart. I watched him closely, looking for a sign. Finally he stood, smiled, and said, "Okay."

"Okay?" Blake and I said in unison.

He told us it would take an hour for the discharge paperwork, and in the meantime he'd ask the nurse to remove the central line. As soon as Wilson was gone, Blake and I locked eyes, smiled, and nodded in unison.

"Let's get out of here before they change their minds," he said, laughing nervously.

"I agree. And you're sure you feel all right."

"I'll be fine, just as soon as we get out of here. I won't believe we're really leaving until we're in the car. Do you have everything packed?"

"I loaded everything before I came. I'm checked out and ready to go."

A few minutes later, the nurse reappeared. "Okay, now sit up, and I'll remove this annoyance," she said. "I would have done it earlier if I'd known you were checking out."

That hour felt like an eternity. We were both afraid they'd find a reason to keep Blake another day, or week. But Wilson finally came back with the completed paperwork, and as he talked, we listened as best we could, and signed where he told us to. When it was over, Wilson shook our hands, wished us well, and continued on his rounds. Soon a woman pushed a wheelchair into the room.

"Mr. Webster?"

"That's me."

"Time to go. We'll stop at the pharmacy downstairs to pick up some of your prescriptions. Meanwhile, your wife can bring the car around and meet us out front."

* * *

As I merged our Pathfinder onto the freeway, heading north to Sonoma County, we both let out a huge sigh of relief. It felt like we had escaped imprisonment, and each mile put us closer to home and freedom. I half expected to see flashing red lights in the rearview mirror. I pictured the cop coming up to the car with the news: "They discharged you by mistake." I noticed Blake glancing behind us, too—two partners in crime.

We'd been told to stop every twenty minutes, so that Blake could get out and stretch his legs to prevent blood clots. Instead, we adjusted his seat so that he could easily move and flex his calf and thigh muscles. Before we left, I had him slip on the chest hugger vest (a strapped adjustable vest worn like a harness) provided by the hospital. It has two front handles that squeeze together to alleviate chest soreness during coughs, sneezes, or routine movement. He also hugged his green flowered heart pillow for extra security.

Bay Area traffic was surprisingly light, and at four o'clock we pulled into the CVS pharmacy's parking lot in Santa Rosa.

"Why don't you stay here," I suggested. "I'll drop off the prescriptions and be right back."

"No, I want to walk some. I'll come in with you."

Marta, the pharmacy clerk, recognized Blake, a regular customer. "Hi, Mr. Webster, how are you today?"

Blake smiled weakly. "I've had better days."

The clerk looked at the four prescriptions, one for the narcotic Oxycodone. "These aren't your usual prescriptions. What's going on?"

Blake opened his jacket and showed off his chest hugger. He pointed at his chest and declared, "Open heart surgery. Had it on Friday. Just got released today."

"Oh, you poor man. How do you feel?"

"Spacey and sore as hell."

Anxious to get us home, I interrupted. "The hospital gave us a few days' supply. We'll be back tomorrow to pick these up."

I helped Blake back to the car. He clutched the vest handles as if he were ready to parachute out of an airplane. His eyes were dull, his expression vacant. Thank God home was only minutes away.

As the automatic garage-door opener squeaked to a stop, I turned off the engine and turned to my husband. "Okay, the stairs will be hard, but there's only four. Just take it slow. I'll come around and help you out—don't move yet," I commanded.

I took a deep breath and got out of the car. Standing suddenly, I felt dizzy and had to steady myself for a second. The blood-pressure medicine I take sometimes causes light-headedness. Clutching the door handle, I hesitated. I could see Blake's face through the passenger-side window. His eyes showed impatience and he clutched his chest in pain. *Oh, God, give me strength.*

With my help, Blake made it up the stairs and into the kitchen. Jesse, our greyhound, would spend one more night boarded at the vet, so we made it to the bedroom without a romping dog leading the way.

I led Blake into the bedroom, to his side of our low platform bed. "Okay, now sit down slowly . . . remember, use only your legs." I propped two pillows against the headboard. "Remember how we did it in the hospital. First, sit as close to the pillow as you can, then swing your legs up. We'll try different-size pillows until you're comfortable."

We'd been warned at the hospital that Blake would have a hard time getting comfortable in a regular bed. Our low-level bed made it a little easier for him. For the next ten minutes, I helped Blake with different arrangements of cushions and pillows. The end result was a good one—husband sitting up and relatively pain free.

I unpacked his medications, found the Oxycodone, shook out two tablets, filled his water container with ice water, and administered the pain meds. As he rested, I went to unload the car.

Once outside, I took a moment to regroup. Shouting children were riding their bicycles in circles at the end of our cul-de-sac. I sat down on the front steps and watched. The boys next door were shooting hoops with their friends on a free-standing basket in the driveway. *Oh, to be young again . . . I feel about a hundred years old.*

An airplane buzzed low overhead, about to land at the airport near where I work, a few minutes away. I thought about our last flight, to and from the Canadian Rockies. Then it hit me—it was over. The waiting, the stress, the scheduling, the logistics—all over. Blake was resting in our bed, and the sun's rays were caressing—and healing—my body and soul. I thanked God.

Chapter Eleven
Recovery

Our First Week Home

I awoke Wednesday morning with a cough, stuffy nose, and headache. I usually have good resistance to colds, but figured I'd picked up a virus at the hospital. Blake had dozed fitfully during the night, and his labored breathing concerned me. It was hard to tell if his congestion was part of his heart and lung problem or just a cold. I worried that if he caught something, it would complicate his recovery. I would bring it up with Dr. Erickson today.

Groggy, stuffed up, and sleep deprived, I took two squirts of my bedside decongestant and shuffled down the hallway to the bathroom. The face greeting me in the mirror had puffy eyes, red-tinged nose, and stringy hair. *C'mon, woman! You gotta pull it together. Not the time to get sick—Blake needs you.*

I managed to clean myself up enough to fake a cheery disposition, then tiptoed back to Blake's side. The cold medicine cleared my nose and took away the headache. I looked down on my sleeping husband and thought about younger days, when we first met. He was so adorable back then with his full beard, long hair, and mustache—he took my breath away. Now beardless, with a peppery gray mustache, and thinning hair, he remained the love of my life—*for better or for worse.*

Blake suddenly rolled over on his back and let out a pirate-like "Aargh." Each eye opened separately. "What time is it?" he mumbled.

"Eight o'clock. How do you feel?" How many times had I asked that in the past few months?

"Stiff and sore."

"We need to be at the Coumadin clinic by nine-thirty, and then our appointment with Dr. Erickson at ten. Can you get out of bed?"

"Yeah . . . I think so."

"Do you need help?"

"No, I think I can do it. You go ahead and get breakfast. I'll call you if I need you."

Blake's resolve to do things on his own, though admirable, was premature. I stayed by his side as he lifted himself from bed. As I started the shower and adjusted the water temperature, he took his morning medications: the beta-blocker, Cardival; the anti-arrhythmia drug, Amiodarone; the diuretic, Triamterene; the painkiller, Oxycocone; and two milligrams of Coumadin. As he got in the shower, he insisted I leave; he could do it himself.

In the kitchen, as I made us both toast and coffee I kept one ear tuned for any unusual sounds from the other room. Soon I heard the electric toothbrush, then the hairdryer. Ten minutes later, a clean, combed, and fully dressed Blake emerged from the bedroom, looking amazingly put together.

Dr. Erickson and the Coumadin Clinic

The Coumadin clinic at Santa Rosa Blood and Heart Monitoring is located on the third floor of the Doyle Park Drive Medical Center. Conveniently for his patients, Dr. Erickson's office is located down the hall on the same floor. Blake and I approached a small table with ten sequentially numbered electronic pagers set in plastic cups. The sign above the table read, "Coumadin Clinic. Take the next sequentially numbered pager and have a seat in the lobby. If all ten pagers are available, walk right in."

"They all seem to be here, so I guess we just go in," I said.

Blake took a minute to answer. He stared at the table. "I don't understand," he said.

"Well, all the beepers seem to be here. See, here's number one. None of the ten are missing, so no one's before us. We can go right in."

Blake stared some more. His medications had slowed his ability to process. Before I could explain further, the door opened. "Hi." A young man in a white medical coat smiled at us. "C'mon in. You're my first patient today."

"Can I come, too?" I asked.

"Oh sure . . . no problem."

The technician escorted us a few steps down the hall and

into a tiny room. He directed Blake to one chair, and I sat in another. The man settled into a seat at his computer and opened a new program. Blake's information popped up on the screen.

"I see that this is your first visit. Dr. Erickson has requested that you maintain a Target INR (International Normalized Ratio) of 2.0 to 3.0. The numbers tell us how quickly your blood will clot. I'm going to prick your finger for a blood sample. I'll test it while you're here, then we'll adjust your dosage accordingly. Dr. Erickson wants you to come in every week for awhile. He'll let you know if and when you can stop the regimen. You have an appointment with him today?"

"Right after this," I chimed in.

"So, you know about how Vitamin K-rich foods interact with the blood-thinning effects of Coumadin?"

I could see that Blake was struggling to focus, so I took over the conversation. "We watched a video at the hospital, and I have a folder of information, including lists of what to eat."

The technician looked at me, but then addressed Blake. "You understand the dietary precautions?"

"I can't eat lots of leafy green vegetables?" Blake asked.

"You can eat them, but stay consistent. If you normally eat lots of salads and green vegetables, that's fine. But don't suddenly eat a plate of broccoli if it's not part of your diet. We're trying to maintain an even blood level of vitamin K. Does that make sense?"

"Yeah," was the only word Blake could muster.

I nodded and said, "I've read all the info and I'll make sure we follow the directions."

The technician dripped a drop of Blake's blood onto a paper test strip and passed it into an electronic device. Within seconds he had the results: Blake's INR was 1.10.

"We'll start you with a two-milligram tablets once a day. If it doesn't go up much, we'll change to two tablets per day. That will likely stabilize you at about 2.6. If you go too high—say, 3.6—we'll reduce it to a half a dose two days a week. The numbers can be numbing, but it's the only way to be sure that you don't run into bleeding problems."

Next stop: Dr. Erickson's office. I took a seat in the living-room-like waiting area, while Blake checked in at the front desk.

"Blake!" the receptionist exclaimed. "Good to see you. How'd it go? You look good."

"Well, I'm still here." Blake held his chest as a chuckle emerged; it quickly turned to a grimace.

"Hey, Blake! Welcome back!" It was Dr. Erickson's assistant, Michael; his voice filled the room. "We'll be with you in a few minutes. You look good, man."

Blake came back and eased into the upholstered chair next to me. It felt like we were little kids on our best behavior in Aunt Martha's front parlor. I even squirmed and kicked my feet to relieve tension.

About ten minutes later, Michael reappeared and ushered us into a small exam room. Blake took off his shirt and chatted with Michael about his surgery and hospital stay while he hooked up the electrodes for an EKG. I silently fidgeted in my chair, still not comfortable as an extra in this drama. A few moments later, Joel Erickson appeared. The routine exam over, he wanted to hear all the gory details. Nothing makes a cardiologist happier than a fresh specimen.

I looked at my watch as doctor, patient, and assistant gossiped about open-heart surgery like it was the latest designer procedure. Each time Blake paused, Joel would say something like, "Oh yeah? And then what happened?" Finally we got to the real reason we were there—Blake's Atrial Fibrillation and what, if anything, to do about it.

"Well, you're still in A-fib," Joel said, pointing at the monitor screen. "See these squiggly lines on the screen and the uneven spacing between beats? That means your heart is fluttering between irregular beats. We'll give it a few weeks. If it doesn't stop on its own, we'll have to shock it."

"Shock it?" Blake said.

"It's called Cardioversion. We can have your device intentionally shock you here in the office, or we can do it at the hospital with external defibrillator paddles. Your choice."

"Do you put me out?" Blake asked. I noticed his eyes dim, brow furl, and his grip tighten on the exam table. I thought I saw tears welling up in his eyes.

Joel laughed. "It's no big deal. You've been shocked before."

"Not while conscious," Blake mumbled.

Joel's expression softened, and in a soothing tone he said, "We'll check you into the hospital for the day and do it there under anesthesia—enough to knock you out, like when you had your ICD replaced. You'll be in and out in a few hours. A simple procedure . . . really."

"So when will we do it?" I asked, thinking about my work schedule. "I plan to go back to work by January 31. If it's after that I'll need to ask for more time off."

"I'll have Tia schedule an appointment for the beginning of March. That will buy us some time to see if the A-fib stops on its own. You'll come in here first, the day of the procedure. If the EKG still shows fluttering, you'll go across the street to Memorial Hospital and be in and out the same day."

As Dr. Erickson rose from his chair, I remembered Blake's congestion. "One more thing," I said. "I picked up a chest cold at the hospital, and Blake also seems congested. I'm concerned it's not a cold, but something else going on with his heart or lungs. How do we know?"

Joel turned toward Blake. “Well, let me have one more listen.” Blake took the required deep breaths as Joel moved the stethoscope around his chest and back. “Yeah, I think he has a cold. His heart sounds fine and his lungs are clear. Runny nose, sneezing, coughing—all par for the course. Hospitals are risky places. He’ll have to let this one run its course, but it’s not dangerous.”

After our appointment, we made arrangements with Tia for March 2. Joel wouldn’t be in town, but his associate, Dr. Jose Ballesteros, would do the Cardioversion.

I squeezed Blake’s hand as we left the office. “In another month or two this will all be over,” I promised.

Steps to Recovery

By January 31, I was back at work. Blake no longer needed constant attention, and my head cold had finally cleared. My ten-minute commute to work made it easy to drive home for lunch to check on my patient. I looked forward to being out of the nursing business, to reestablishing a normal routine.

At home, Blake was bored and restless. Our dog Jesse required two daily walks, so they got out of the house mornings and afternoons. Despite that exercise, Blake continued to have a difficult time sleeping. It was hard to get comfortable lying on his back, propped up by cushions and pillows. He tried to work, and did manage to complete some routine tasks, but he couldn’t sit for long at the computer. The five medications fogged his mind and limited his creativity. I observed his growing frustration as I tried to keep us both on an even emotional keel. Some evenings found us both in tears, each trying to comfort the other; we were physically and mentally exhausted. Yet, going through this together brought us closer. Though we tried to take one day at a time, the crisis cemented our resolve to continue to move forward.

Thirty days after surgery, we made the final trip to PCCVS in Redwood City for Blake's follow-up appointment with RN Sylvia Beach. After an hour-long appointment, we were reassured that recovery was on schedule. All we needed to do was stay with the program.

Our checklist included:

- Pain Medicine. Stop the Oxycodone. A patient on any narcotic shouldn't drive, and Blake was anxious to regain his independence. Sylvia recommended he substitute two 325-milligram tablets of regular strength Tylenol every eight hours to start. Then as the pain subsided, he should reduce the dosage to two tablets once per day, then one tablet per day until he felt comfortable enough to stop altogether.
- Keep moving. Maintain a balance between walking, sitting, and lying down. It's recommended that you not spend full days in the bedroom, lest muscles atrophy. It is psychologically and physically beneficial to stay in the living areas of your home. Be aware that you continue to be susceptible to blood clots, especially in the legs. Don't sit for more than forty-five minutes at a time, and don't cross your legs. Start a walking regimen of at least two walks a day. Begin with ten minutes at a

time and increase incrementally to thirty minutes twice a day.

▪ Continue your breathing exercises. Use the larger inspirometer (the same one given to you at the hospital) at least five to six times daily.

▪ Lifting. For the first month, do not lift, push, or pull more than five pounds. After sixty days this can be increased to ten pounds. Then give it another month before you try twenty to twenty-five pounds. It's better to be careful than to risk further injury to your rib cage and chest muscles. You may hear clicking sounds in the breastbone area. This is normal. Your ribs have been wired to facilitate healing of the broken bones. The sound will remind you to not do too much too soon with your upper body.

▪ Incision care. Check your incisions daily. It's fine to wash with gentle soap and water. After showering, pat the area dry with a fresh towel. If you notice an increase in redness, swelling, or oozing of the incision, call the surgeon's office immediately. The incision area will appear plump at first—this is normal. Be sure to protect it from the sun, since this is new skin that burns easily. Numbness in the area is also normal; regular feeling will return over time.

▪ Itching. Your skin may be dry because of soaps used at the hospital or as a reaction to medications. Moisturing lotions are helpful as long as they aren't applied to the incision area. Call your family physician if the sensation becomes unbearable.

▪ Excessive perspiration. Even in the absence of a fever, sensations of hot and cold may come and go. It's not unusual to perspire more when asleep. Your body will return to normal over time.

▪ Tension release. Continue with simple stretching exercises; be aware of your posture when you sit and stand. Some patients find that a heating pad set on low relaxes tight areas; however, don't place it on your incision.

▪ Concentration. For Blake this was the biggest challenge. He wanted to get back to work as soon as possible. Since he works at home on his computer, he thought he could immediately pick up where he left off—an unrealistic goal. As the patient is weaned from medications and the body heals, normal mental activity will return. Give it time. It's frustrating, but it will get better.

▪ Constipation. Pain medication slows bowel movement. Adjust your diet to include more fiber. Eat fresh fruits, vegetable, and whole grains. Drink at least six to eight glasses of water per day. Warm tea or broth is helpful. Take a gentle laxative at bedtime, as required.

▪ Sleep. Regular sleep patterns will be the last thing to return to normal. Take your pain medicine thirty minutes before retiring. Try to avoid naps during the day. Walk and exercise until pleasantly fatigued; adjust pace and distance if exhausted at the end of the day. You should be sleeping with your head elevated for two to four months.

▪ Emotional ups and downs. Feelings of helplessness, vulnerability, sadness, and depression are a natural result of the trauma you've been though. Some days will be better than others. Allow the feelings out without wallowing in them. Be kind to yourself. You've been through a lot. If you feel overwhelmed and it's not getting better, call your primary-care physician for a therapist referral.

▪ Miscellaneous changes. Some perceived feelings are hard to pinpoint or describe. Each patient's body is unique, and unexpected reactions may occur. For instance, some people have blurry vision after surgery. Don't call your eye doctor until after recovery. More than likely your eyes will return to normal in a month or two.

▪ Call your surgeon if: a) you're running a fever, b) your incision is inflamed and increasingly painful, c) you feel or hear frequent grinding or popping in your chest area, or d) your legs become numb or painful.

▪ Call your cardiologist if: a) you feel a fast or irregular heartbeat, b) you're easily winded, c) you're dizzy and lightheaded, d) your weight has increased more than two pounds overnight or five pounds in a week, or e) your legs are swollen.

Caregiver's checklist for the first 30-60 days.

▪ Stay in the present. Deal with each challenge as it appears. Don't fret about the future.

▪ Keep worry to a minimum. The bills, work concerns, and lifestyle changes will all be dealt with in due time. Address these issues as they become a reality, not before. You'll be amazed at how well things will work out once you and your patient are past recovery.

▪ Relationship problems. Don't expect your patient to be himself (or herself) for several months. Learn to deflect negative remarks with a shrug and a hug. If after a month depression is still an issue for either of you, seek professional help. But don't despair.

▪ Try to stay positive. You are the patient's "rock" to lean on. Try not to nag, preach, hover, or scold your patient. Your positive attitude contributes to quick recovery.

▪ Care for yourself. Caregiver's Syndrome is a common reaction. Recognize the symptoms of stress, fear, loneliness, guilt, anger, fatigue, self doubt, and depression. As always, find time for yourself; solicit help and do the things you enjoy as much as possible.

▪ Stay active during recovery. Continue to attend doctor's visits and ask questions. Having the facts will alleviate worry.

▪ Normalize life. Make every attempt to return to normal. Get yourself and the patient out of the house. As soon as possible see friends and family. Go back to work.

▪ Eat well. Begin dietary changes you've been putting off. Cook, eat, and enjoy the foods that are good for your patient. They are good for you, too.

▪ Join a support group, like Mended Hearts. Human contact with others who share your challenges is a blessing.

Chapter Twelve
Full Circle

Outpatient Cardioversion

We drove in silence to the Doyle Park Medical Building for what seemed like the hundredth EKG. Michael conducted the routine test, looked at Blake, and said, "It looks like you're going across the street."

"Across the street" meant that Blake's heart, still in A-fib, needed its first intentionally administered shock. We had hoped Blake's heart would return to a normal rhythm on its own, but no such luck. Tia had scheduled an Outpatient Cardioversion at Memorial Hospital for early afternoon. I didn't bother moving the car; we walked to the main lobby and Admissions.

The afternoon lobby traffic, unlike our prior early-morning check-ins, bustled. We settled near the reception desk, where white-haired matronly volunteers answered questions and directed visitors. We almost didn't hear our name called above the din.

"Webster? Blake Webster?" the admittance clerk called out.

"We're here," Blake called back.

It took me a few seconds to gather my laptop, purse, and jacket. Blake, already seated in the clerk's cubicle when I arrived, answered the standard questions one more time. I didn't bother to sit down. The clerk had attached the obligatory wrist bands, and I knew we'd be on our way in no time. I stepped aside as an orderly came up behind me with a wheelchair and Blake got in. I padded along after them, thinking I needed to switch to a lighter computer; my shoulder ached from all the schlepping I'd done in the past sixty days.

The orderly pointed me toward a small waiting room. "You can wait in here." I recognized it as the same one I'd been in when they replaced Blake's first ICD unit and again for Blake's last angiogram before surgery. "We'll be back for you after he's prepped."

I settled into a corner chair, next to the brochure rack. Colorful pamphlet covers showed pictures of smiling faces of doctors and patients, obviously glad to be giving and receiving the best of care. I was way past believing that any of this could be fun. As I booted my computer, I was glad, however, to find that the Wi-Fi signal was fast and strong. My laptop was my best buddy, my link to the outside world. Well, second-best buddy.

I glanced at the TV—sound on low—tuned to local news and weather. The family seated across from me discussed their husband and father's latest bypass operation, between chatter about where they should eat dinner. They, like me, had sat in this room more than once.

A half hour later, a nurse cracked the door, looked in my direction, and asked, "Elaine Webster?"

"That's me."

* * *

Cardioversion, a simple procedure that takes less than thirty minutes, occupied most of our afternoon. Once again, I sat next to Blake's bed in the short-stay unit. As he was poked and prodded, I silently hoped this would be our last hospital visit. Dr. Ballesteros gave Blake a short-acting deep sedation before he externally shocked the heart through attached electrodes. I wasn't allowed to watch, but I stayed close by before and after the procedure.

While I waited for Blake to wake up, the doctor pulled me aside. "Is he always this hard to put under?" he asked.

"I don't know. I never thought about it, why?"

"I gave him the sedative equivalent of half a bottle of scotch before I could start. I've never had a patient require so much sedation, so I want you to be especially careful when you get home. He may want to go to sleep for the night."

"Well, I'll keep an eye on him, but I'll be surprised if that happens. It's got something to do with Webster willpower, I guess. They are always in control." I laughed alone.

I was right. Blake couldn't wait to get out of there. He tolerated the required wheelchair and slipped into the Pathfinder without assistance. As I pulled away from the patient loading zone he asked me, "So, what's for dinner?"

After Cardioversion report any of the following to your cardiologist:

- Irritation, blistering, or soreness in chest area
- Dizziness, confusion, lightheadedness
- Heart palpitations or irregular heartbeat
- Difficulty breathing
- Nausea or vomiting
- Sharp chest pains or pains in your arm
- Abdominal pain
- Blood in the urine
- Change in vision or speech
- Trouble walking or using your limbs
- Drooping facial muscles or eyelids

A Clean Bill of Health

I plopped down at the kitchen table and put my feet up. Jesse, our greyhound, nuzzled his nose under my arm, and I absentmindedly rubbed his ears.

Blake poured two glasses of Zinfandel and handed one to me. He sat across the table.

"So, how'd it go at Erickson's today?" I asked. It had been three months since Blake's surgery and six weeks since the cardioversion. He'd had a follow-up appointment with his cardiologist that morning.

"It went great. Michael did an EKG, and the A-fib hasn't come back yet. The best part is I don't have to take Coumadin any more."

I set my glass down, pushed the dog aside, and took a deep breath. "So, you're off all the medications except for Coreg?" I could barely believe it. The constant trips to the pharmacy, the lightheadedness, the absent look in my husband's eyes were behind us. I looked at the calendar. "You know our anniversary is next week?" I smiled mischievously. "I put in for the week off work . . . wanna go somewhere? We could go look at the ocean from some hotel room and drink champagne."

"Well, it's funny you say that. I called the Breaker's Inn when I got home from the doctor's. We have reservations for Tuesday night. How's that sound?"

The Breaker's Inn is the ocean-front hotel where Blake's medical journey began. It was from there, twelve years ago, that we called Dr. Devore's office in a panic after Blake's first major episode. Not wanting to relive those days, we hadn't been back; now it seemed right to go. We had come full circle, and a celebration was in order.

I reached across the table and squeezed Blake's hand. "Sounds great. In fact it sounds wonderful."

Thirty-Seventh Wedding Anniversary

The rooms at the Breaker's Inn have names. The Normandy Room, decorated with French antiques and art prints, was where we cut our twenty-fifth anniversary short. With the haunting memory of Blake tossing all night in the frilly four-poster bed, we decided on a different room. On April 19, 2011, I swiped the hotel card key to the San Francisco-themed room instead. As I pushed open the door, a sunny glow reflected off the tan walls and high vaulted ceiling.

"Do you believe we're here?" I asked. I wondered if I should pinch myself; that's what they say you should do when something's too good to be true. Tears welled in my eyes and a lump filled my throat. Blake set the overnight case on the small sofa facing the fireplace and gazed out on the ocean, speechless.

"Do you remember when we first met?" Blake asked. I nodded and he put his arm around my waist. "You served me lentil soup and we went to your meditation group that evening."

"Yeah, and Richard, the leader, gave you the third degree. He was sure you were trying to take advantage of me."

"Well, I was." Blake chuckled lasciviously and drew me closer. We stood there for what felt like an hour, holding each other, gazing at the ocean, taking it all in. At one point, I began to cry. Not the huge sobs I'd let flow in Redwood City, but gentle tears of joy and relief. I knew at that moment that I had my husband back.

Blake—Better Than Ever

Blake's leaky valve resulted from several serious child-hood illnesses in the 1950s, including rheumatic fever. The doctors told his parents that his murmur would cause heart complications later in life, and those problems developed as expected.

Now, each day since surgery has brought renewed strength and spirit. It's been six months and Blake's never felt better. Sure, there's still some soreness, but essentially he's experiencing full recovery. What was once a death sentence is now, through modern medical technology, a rebirth. Once you've decided that a surgical option is the right decision, know that afterwards, life will be better than ever for you and your loved one.

Postrecovery Guidelines

As an active health partner, review the following list of postrecovery guidelines with your patient.

- Stick with your diet regimen. Continue to eat as outlined in the previous chapters—fresh, wholesome, and low sodium.
- Stay active. This is more important than ever as we age. Maintain a healthy weight. Strength-train to minimize bone loss and maximize muscle balance. Condition your core muscles with yoga and/or pilates to maintain flexibility and balance. Get plenty of cardiovascular exercise: bike, hike, swim, play sports—whatever activities you enjoy.
- Adjust physical activity to your fitness level. If you've never exercised before, take it slow and make steady progress. Check with your cardiologist and primary-care physician before you start. And remember that heat can be hard on your heart. Take precautionary measures, especially if you continue to take beta-blockers, diuretics, ace inhibitors, or calcium channel blockers. All these medications exaggerate the body's response to heat. Exercise with a friend or around other people. Join a

health club or your local YMCA. Wear lightweight breathable fabrics and drink enough water. Take regular breaks. Seek immediate medical attention if you have symptoms of heat exhaustion or heatstroke.

Signs of heat exhaustion: Headaches, profuse sweating, chills, dizziness, muscle cramps, rapid shallow breathing, nausea, vomiting.

Signs of heatstroke: Warm dry skin without sweating, rapid pulse, mental confusion, loss of consciousness, high fever, throbbing headaches, nausea, vomiting.

▪ Be careful in cold temperatures, which can contribute to heart-disease risk factors. Cold weather constricts blood vessels and raises blood pressure. This and the medications you take may make it hard for your body to handle low temperatures. Activities like downhill and cross-country skiing should not be part of your exercise routine without your doctor's consent. Low oxygen levels at high elevations increase the heart rate as your body tries to compensate. Cross-country skiing relies on upper body strength, which can boost blood pressure and increase risk for a heart attack.

▪ See life as a gift, a new beginning. Make an effort to try new things. Make new friends. Mental stimulation is as important as physical activity.

▪ Right the wrongs in your life. If addictive behavior or substance abuse contributed to your heart problems, work a twelve-step program tailored to your needs. You will find the support and friendship you need for full recovery. Make amends to those you've hurt.

- Adopt an attitude of self-acceptance and self-love. Take a moment to focus on your attributes. Make a list and carry it with you for daily review.
- Keep good company. Associate with people that affirm you. Stay away from those who make you feel small and/or inadequate. Stand up for yourself, learn to say no, walk away from abuse, and don't apologize when you've done nothing wrong. When people try and drag you down and you don't have the option to leave (as in work environments), learn to filter out inappropriate criticism. Don't take it too seriously.
- No one is perfect; don't expect yourself to be. You are unique with special talents, so stop comparing yourself to others. Be creative—use existing talents to their fullest and pursue new ideas.
- Find God, in whatever way makes sense to you.
- Maintain a close relationship with your medical providers. Follow your doctor's advice and check-up schedule.
- Take all medications as prescribed. Purchase a pill organizer from your local pharmacy. These plastic boxes are designed to hold from one week's to one month's worth of prescriptions. There are slots for morning, noon, and night. The system helps you track what to take and when. It also alerts you to refill schedules. Keep a list of current medications with you at all times. You'll need this information for doctor visits and for paramedics in an emergency.

Chapter Thirteen
Mind, Body, and Soul Food

Keep it Simple

As a heart patient you must pay extra attention to your diet. What an awful word, diet. As it rolls off our tongue, every cell in our body says, *No, I don't want to change . . . I don't want give up all that's dear to me . . . all that comfort, joy, and deliciousness . . . I can't diet the rest of my life . . . I'd rather die.*

Well, the good news is that you need not suffer. You can now live, love, and enjoy life with relative abandon. And you're not going to die, at least not soon. Isn't that why you fought through surgery and recovery? You are alive, well, and soon to be better than ever.

In the kitchen, think fresh and simple. Cooking, eating, and enjoying food is easy. Stop trying to complicate it by spending hours in pursuit of the perfect meal. When you sit down at the table to eat, be thankful for the feast set before you. Look at it, love it, and above all else taste it—really taste it. It's a gift.

Getting Through the Work Week

Blake and I are busy people, and busy people are most productive when they're organized. If you have children, you face extra challenges. If they're old enough, solicit their help; you will teach them valuable skills. They have learned about heart disease first hand; now they can contribute to the family's healthy lifestyle, a lifestyle that will carry over into their adulthood.

Prepare weekly menus and pick a day for grocery shopping. Buy foods that the entire family can eat, including the heart patient. Emphasize that natural, low-salt foods are best for everyone. Divide meal preparation among family members, and have all ingredients available in your well-stocked kitchen. Utilize every kitchen gadget available to prepare quality, low-cost, tasty, and simple meals.

Most mornings the typical family flies haphazardly out of the house with little time for breakfast. Keep the refrigerator stocked with healthy grab-and-go foods. Yogurt, fruit, eight-ounce containers of low-fat or soy milk, and energy bars are all good choices. Send the family off with pre-packed lunch coolers, and give them enough food to get them through the day. Send children to school with healthy in-between-meal snacks, to keep them away from the salt- and sugar-laden junk in vending machines. Adults seeking healthy lifestyle changes should pack well-thought-out meals the night before—another argument for weekly menus and organized shopping trips. Once again, simplicity is key, but pack what you and your family like as you watch calories, fat, and salt content.

Teach love through food. Whether you are single, or part of a couple or family, nothing is more nurturing than food preparation. The world is full of egoists and narcissists—the self-consumed. They don't realize that providing for others returns multiple rewards, in the kitchen and in life. If you live alone, volunteer at your local food kitchen or organize potluck dinners with friends. It will do your heart good. As a couple, celebrate your commitment to each other with a delicious meal. As a family, make dinner quality time.

Basic guidelines for teaching kids to cook:

- Hands-on adult supervision for young children ages seven to eleven is essential. Older children, twelve to thirteen, should have an adult nearby to assist and advise when necessary. Teenagers usually have no problem going it alone, especially if they grew up cooking.
- Teach your children basic kitchen safety. Show them how to properly hold and use sharp knifes, clean cutting surfaces, use oven mitts, and set oven temperatures and burner levels.
- Keep measuring spoons and cups stored at child level. It's fun for children if one kitchen drawer holds all their favorite utensils. As with their toys, it's important that they learn what is theirs, where it belongs, and how to clean up after they're done.
- To avoid frustration with botched recipes, match the task to the age and abilities of each child.

Two favorite children's recipes:

"I'll skewer, you heat the barbeque, Kabobs"

For the Kabobs:
2 lbs. boneless, skinless chicken thighs cut into 1-inch cubes
2 bell peppers, diced into large pieces
1 large onion chunked
2 pints cherry tomatoes
2 pints mushrooms with stalks removed

For the Marinade:
½ cup balsamic vinegar
½ cup olive oil
2 tablespoons prepared mustard
2 tablespoons minced garlic
Freshly ground black pepper to taste

An hour or two before dinner, place the first set of ingredients in a glass or ceramic bowl. Mix the second set of ingredients and pour them over the first. Cover the mixture and refrigerate. At dinnertime an adult prepares the grill. Charcoal should be allowed to burn down to glowing grey coals. Gas barbeques should be set on medium. During the preheat the child pushes the meat and vegetables in random succession onto the skewers. The adult lays the skewers on the grill, turning frequently until cooked through. Round out the meal with rice and cold watermelon. Serves four.

"Ground Turkey Tacos"

For the filling:

1 pound ground turkey
Juice two limes
¼ cup fresh chopped cilantro
1 tablespoon Salt Free Fajita Seasoning
(See resource section in Chapter 14)
2 tablespoons water

For the toppings:

2 large avocados mashed into a thick paste
Juice of one lemon
Touch of Tabasco to taste
1 head iceberg lettuce
2 fresh tomatoes
1 eight-ounce brick of cheese

Hand-mix the filling; cook over medium heat in a large skillet until the meat is well done. To make the guacamole, mix the first three ingredients together and set aside. Shred iceberg lettuce with a food processor or grater. (Depending on the child's age, this may require adult assistance.) Chop the tomatoes by hand and shred the cheese. Serve buffet-style, each topping in a separate bowl, allowing diners to build their own tacos. I use prepared taco shells, which I heat briefly in the microwave. (Read the labels—some have no salt.) Serve with chili on the side. (Look for no-salt canned chili.) Serves four to six.

Or prepare *Blake's Favorite Crock Pot Chili*. Blake cooks the way he works: Use logic, be prepared, have everything you need, do it early, do it fast, let it simmer, and relish the results. Accordingly, he makes his favorite dinners in a slow cooker.

"Blake's Favorite Crock Pot Chili"

2 cans no-salt pinto beans
2 cans diced tomatoes with jalapenos
2 cloves chopped garlic
1 small chopped onion
1 medium bell pepper chopped
1 teaspoon chili powder
¼ teaspoon cayenne pepper
½ teaspoon cumin
1 teaspoon dried basil
¼ teaspoon crushed red pepper

Early in the day, throw everything into the slow cooker in no particular order. Set the dial to low and walk away. Blake brags that he can put this meal together in ten minutes, including clean-up. All I know is that when I walk in the door after work, the house smells wonderful. Serves six.

Weekend Extravaganza

As with many families, our kitchen is central to our home life. It's a place to plan, discuss, debate, share hugs, and some days even cry. It's where comfort food and friendship reign supreme. We do our best thinking and planning sitting at the kitchen table.

On the weekends I especially like to cook. One meal in particular conjures up visions of a rustic gathering of friends and family on a sunny hillside in France—Chicken Cassoulet. Served with crusty French bread, it is a complete meal. It can be made with chicken or as a Vegan delight by substituting firm tofu for the meat and using vegetable broth. It can simmer on the stove for hours or be eaten right away. For potlucks and parties, you can toss it in a slow cooker or serve buffet-style in a chafing dish.

“French Country-Style Cassoulet”

Ingredients:

Olive oil
12 boneless chicken thighs cut into pieces
1 cup sliced mushrooms
One diced onion (I sometimes use onion & shallots)
Lots of diced garlic (4 cloves or more to taste)
1 teaspoon dried thyme (I also add whatever fresh herbs look good from the patio: rosemary, savory, chives, but only 1/4 cup or so chopped)
2 bay leaves
2 15-ounce cans salt-free Cannellini Beans, drained & rinsed
1 15-ounce can diced tomatoes with peppers
1 15-ounce can salt-free chicken broth
Fresh ground pepper to taste
Some fresh chopped Italian parsley.

Heat the oil in a large skillet and brown the chicken for 7 to 8 minutes. Add the mushrooms, onion, garlic, thyme, fresh herbs, and bay leaf. Mix well, cover, and cook for 5 to 6 minutes. Add the beans, tomato, broth, and pepper. Bring back to a boil. Reduce heat to low, cover, and simmer gently for 5 minutes. Then keep warm for guests, or just dish into bowls and eat. It’s also good served with some Dijon mustard for dipping the chicken or tofu pieces, and some Tabasco for the spice lovers.

* * *

> *It's so beautifully arranged on the plate,*
> *you know someone's fingers have been all over it.*
> *—Julia Child*

"Let's cook," I said, encircling Blake's neck with my arms and kissing the top of his head.

Blake's hands left the computer keyboard and took hold of mine. "I thought you'd never ask," he said.

Six months after his surgery, I decided it was time to renew the romantic side of our relationship. I'd been grocery shopping, and fresh organic foods covered the kitchen counter. I'd pulled out our best china, set a colorful table for two, arranged a dozen red roses as a centerpiece, and chilled a bottle of Chardonnay wine. Freshly clipped sprigs of rosemary and thyme suffused the air with their aroma.

Blake had been at work all Sunday morning in his office, oblivious to my efforts. Well, I'd fix that.

"Come help me in the kitchen," I cooed.

Blake's hands slid up and down my arms. He swiveled his chair around and pulled me down for a kiss. I pulled him up and led him out of the room, swinging the door shut behind us. No more work today. We stood together at the

the kitchen counter, arms around each others' waists, surveying the cornucopia of ingredients.

Spread out on the counter was everything we needed for a romantic roast chicken dinner for two.

4-pound roasting chicken (plump)
Fresh-cut herbs (one fistful each of rosemary and thyme)
1 large fragrant lemon (ripe and juicy)
Olive oil (local blend infused with tangerines)
1 ½ pounds Yukon Gold potatoes (scrubbed clean)
1 pound green beans (cut into bite-size lengths)
2 tablespoons unsalted butter (a touch of forbidden decadence)
3 tablespoons sliced almonds (our favorite nuts)

"Preheat the oven to 400 degrees," I instructed my partner.

"That's not too hot?" he asked.

"Not for me," I answered in my best bedroom voice.

As Blake peeled the potatoes and cut them into one-inch chunks, I clipped the rosemary with kitchen shears, placed it in a large glass bowl, and mixed in 2 ½ tablespoons of olive oil.

"Are you done with the potatoes?" I asked.

"They're ready. Help me slide them into the bowl."

I held the cutting board as Blake pushed the tubers into the olive oil mixture.

"I'll start on the chicken while you fix the beans," I coached.

I removed the giblets from the chicken's cavity and washed and dried the bird. I packed the empty cavity with the fresh thyme and the whole uncut lemon.

"Help me tie the legs together and tuck the wings—they keep slipping away," I said.

Blake held the appendages in place while I successfully trussed the poultry. We dipped our fingers in a small bowl of olive oil and rubbed it into the plump flesh. After we both washed our hands, I placed the chicken on a rack in the roasting pan and lowered it into the preheated oven.

"We have a half hour before we need to do anything else. Got any ideas?" I queried with a wink.

"One or two . . . "

* * *

Back in the kitchen, we leisurely finished meal preparation. Blake spread a half tablespoon of olive oil on a rimmed baking sheet. He placed the marinated potatoes on top and spread them evenly around the pan. He brushed the chicken with more olive oil and then slid the pan of potatoes next to the roast. I filled the bottom of a sauce pan with water, set in a steamer basket full of green beans, and set the burner on high. As the vegetables steamed for ten minutes, I turned the roasting potatoes with a spatula, and added butter to a large skillet over a medium heat. To the melted butter I added the sliced almonds and sautéed them. Once they had some color, (approximately two minutes), I lifted the bean-filled steamer rack from the adjacent saucepan and carefully slid the vegetables into the skillet.

An hour and ten minutes after placing the chicken in the oven, Blake uncorked the wine to let it breathe. The potatoes, having roasted for thirty-five minutes, were firm yet cooked through when tested with a fork. We kept the green beans warm in their skillet.

As Blake artfully arranged the potatoes and beans on plates, I carved the chicken. We complemented each other perfectly: I enjoy dark meat and Blake prefers the white tender breast. I placed generous portions of each on the appropriate plates, and we sat down to eat.

We paused to say our form of grace. Clinking our glasses of wine, we smiled and said in unison, “Thank you, God.”

Chapter Fourteen
Resource Guide

Author's Information

Elaine Webster
P.O. Box 3153
Santa Rosa, CA 95402
Elaine@mediadesign-mds.com

Other Books by Elaine Webster

Jesse's Tale: Overcoming Fear Aggression and Separation Anxiety in an Adopted Greyhound

Suggested Reading

Heart Healthy Cookbooks

American Heart Association: Low-Salt Cookbook
Clarkson Potter/Publishers, New York

The No-Salt, Lowest-Sodium, Light Meals Book
Donald A Gazzaniga and Maureen A Gazzaniga

Healthy Heart Cookbook
Edith Tibbetts and Karen Cadwell, Ph.D., R.N.

The No-Salt Cookbook
David C. Anderson and Thomas D. Anderson

Food Content Guides

The Complete Book of Food Counts
Corinne T. Netzer

Pocket Guide to Low Sodium Foods
Bobbie Mostyn

Low-Sodium Product Sources

Healthy Heart Market Online Store: The Leading Source for Low and No Sodium Food Products
http://healthyheartmarket.com/

The Spice Hunter
http://spicehunter.com/

Mrs. Dash
http://www.mrsdash.com/?s_cid=c3a:google:brand:mrs+dash

Medical Information Websites

American Medical Association
http://www.ama-assn.org/

Medline Plus
http://www.nlm.nih.gov/medlineplus/

American College of Cardiology: CardioSource
http://www.cardiosource.org/

Medical Library Association: Deciphering Medspeak
http://www.mlanet.org/resources/medspeak/

American Heart Association
http://www.heart.org/HEARTORG/

Medical Insurance Research and Comparison Websites

The National Committee for Quality Assurance
http://www.ncqa.org/Default.aspx

Consumer Reports:
Health.org
http://www.consumerreports.org/health/insurance/health-insurance.htm

National Association of Insurance Commissioners
https://eapps.naic.org/cis/

eHealthInsurance
http://www.ehealthinsurance.com/

Made in the USA
Lexington, KY
26 July 2017